BI 3391389

CW00794555

BIRMINGHAM CITY
UNIVERSITY
LIBRARY

DISCARDED

18/01/2015

Date
Certified

The Three Dimensions of Stuttering:
Neurology, Behaviour and Emotion

Second Edition

PB

MSL

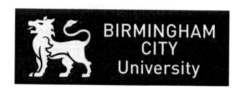

BIRMINGHAM
CITY
University

FOR REFERENCE ONLY

NOT TO BE
TAKEN AWAY

The Three Dimensions of Stuttering: Neurology, Behaviour and Emotion

Second Edition

Robert Logan

The University of Central Arkansas
Conway, Arkansas

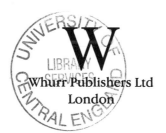

Whurr Publishers Ltd
London

© 1999 Whurr Publishers Ltd
Second edition published 1999
by Whurr Publishers Limited
19b Compton Terrace, London N1 2UN, England
First edition published by Pro-Ed, Austin, Texas

Reprinted 1999

All rights reserved. No part of this publication may be
reproduced, stored in a retrieval system, or transmitted
in any form or by any means, electronic, mechanical,
photocopying, recording or otherwise, without the prior
permission of Whurr Publishers Limited.

This publication is sold subject to the conditions that it
shall not, by way of trade or otherwise, be lent, resold,
hired out, or otherwise circulated without the
publisher's prior consent in any form of binding or
cover other than that in which it is published and
without a similar condition including this condition
being imposed upon any subsequent purchaser.

British Library Cataloguing in Publication Data
A catalogue record for this book is available from the
British Library.

ISBN 1 86156 073 7

UNIVERSITY OF
CENTRAL ENGLAND

Book no. 33913897

Subject no. R616.8554091 Log

LIBRARY SERVICES

Printed and bound in the UK by Athenæum Press Ltd,
Gateshead, Tyne & Wear.

Contents

Preface to the second edition   vii

Acknowledgements   ix

Introduction   1

Chapter 1   7

Neurophysiological review

Chapter 2   49

Conditioning and stuttering

Chapter 3   61

Neuroimaging studies of stuttering

Chapter 4   81

Diagnostics

Chapter 5   86

Treatment

Afterword   96

Appendix: Connections of the amygdala   99

References   107

Index   113

Preface to the second edition

It is wonderful to be able to write a second edition of this text. There have been remarkable research reports since the first edition and I am grateful to be able to present them and to incorporate them into the limbic model. Those of you who read the earlier edition will find this one very different in both style and content. The perspective of several years has pointed out to me how stilted, formal and, well . . . pompous the writing style was in the first edition. I have made every effort to avoid such errors here. I hope you find this edition both informative and at times amusing.

The contents have been greatly altered. The review of brain structures and areas in Chapter One has been improved and expanded. Information on the basal ganglia and the cerebellum is included that strongly suggests that these areas contribute not just to speech and language but also to cognition and emotional expression. I think many of you will be surprised by the larger role assigned to these areas for responsibilities not traditionally associated with them.

Chapter Two is entirely new and describes the acquisition process of conditioned responses and how such responses can interfere with normal motor initiation and completion. Chapter Three is also new and reviews the findings of several of the most recent imaging studies of the brains of subjects who stutter. The results of each study are viewed through the perspective of the information presented in the review in Chapter One and the data on learning and conditioning in Chapter Two. Chapter Four addresses the ways in which the information in the previous chapters can be used diagnostically. Chapter Five presents treatment goals and procedures distilled from the first four chapters. It also attempts to summarize the main thrust of the information and inference presented in a section entitled – what else? – 'summary'. Finally, there is an 'afterword' that suggests some questions and activities for future research.

I very much hope that this second edition results in controversy and that you enjoy it. I hope that it stimulates your interest in the limbic system, the neocerebellum, basal ganglia and the right hemisphere and how these areas and structures may contribute to both the etiology and maintenance of stuttering. There is an answer to the why and how of stuttering – we just haven't asked the right questions yet. I hope that this text contributes a few good questions and, maybe, one or two answers . . .

Acknowledgements

I want to take this opportunity to thank the following people for their help, inspiration, understanding, patience and overall forgivingness in the development of this manuscript:

Susan Moss-Logan for her unflagging belief in my abilities (particularly impressive in light of my many deficits).
Chad Nye for his encouragement and many kindnesses over the years.
Avery O Vaughn for his wise counsel and instruction in the field of neuro-physiology.
LL Schendel for his wise counsel and support.
The faculty of audiology and speech pathology at Florida State University.
James Thurman for all of his support over the years here at the University of Central Arkansas.
Kim Rogers, research assistant and juggler, for her patience and ability to keep several assignments spinning successfully in the air at the same time.
James Montegue, Professor, University of Arkansas, Little Rock, for his support, his review of the manuscript, and for his encouragement throughout my career at UCA.

Introduction

The etiology of stuttering is not known and may well never be known. As has been said by others, stuttering may have as many etiologies as there are people who stutter. This is not to say that it is not profitable to explore the issue of etiology here; brain mechanisms have to be at work and it would be very profitable, from both prevention and treatment standpoints, to identify these mechanisms. The question of the etiology of stuttering undoubtedly underscores the old 'nature/nurture' argument concerning explanations for behaviour. The answer to the question of whether stuttering is caused by either of these seemingly different perspectives is: 'yes'. This might appear to be no answer but genetic studies reviewed later in this book point out that only the *predisposition* to stutter is passed down, not the actual speech characteristic. The individual, usually male, must have this predisposition triggered by the environment for the stuttering to emerge. It seems reasonable to assume that if the environment targeted some behaviour other than speech another result might emerge – for instance, spastic colitis.

It is this uncertainty about the etiology (-gies?) of the disorder that should cause researchers to pause before they claim to have discovered 'the' etiology of stuttering. At this point in our ability to investigate, it is far better (and safer) to claim to have identified some of the brain mechanisms involved in this disorder. Identifying these areas presents enough of a challenge given the current state of research methodology. Claims to have discovered the etiology of the complex disorder of stuttering should always be viewed with scepticism.

Etiology aside, the search for the cause of the underlying speech characteristics associated with stuttering has enjoyed a controversial and fascinating history. Beginning with Orton and Travis's 'lack of cerebral dominance' hypothesis in the early part of the century (1929), the history of the search presents a circuitous route that has mirrored the *Zeitgeist* of the generations of researchers through which the search passed. Early unsophisticated neurophysiology, blood sugar levels, psychoanalysis, behaviourism and various eclectic theories drawing from some or all of

1

these earlier approaches have reflected the collective wisdom of those times and the then-accepted explanations of human behaviour.

In 1931, Orton and Travis (1929) suggested that stuttering was the result of neither cerebral hemisphere exerting dominance over the other so far as cranial nerve control of speech musculature is concerned. This lack of dominance resulted in instructions from the central nervous system reaching the two halves of the speech system at different times, presumably with different commands concerning speed, accuracy, velocity and range of speech movements. The resulting aberrant movements were considered to be the underlying cause of the characteristic behaviours associated with stuttering. In 1996, a research team led by Fox and the Ingrams, using positron emission tomography, reported right cerebral hemisphere dominance in subjects who stuttered but a return to more normal left-hemisphere dominance during induced fluency tasks. This team also found other intriguing data to be reviewed later but the aim here is to suggest that neurophysiological explanations of stuttering behaviour are once more in favour.

The return to this line of enquiry that has been made possible by the development of increasingly sophisticated non-invasive imaging techniques should not be misunderstood as minimizing contributions from other perspectives that have attempted to explain stuttering. Just as stuttering does not exist in a neurophysiological void, neither does the disorder exist in an emotional/psychological or learning void. Genetic studies suggest that only the predisposition to stutter may be passed on; it is the environment that triggers this predisposition and results in stuttering. In order for the trigger to be pulled the child must experience some (presumably negative) emotional/psychological speech-based impact from the environment. Further, this negative reaction to speaking must, of course, be learned by the child. Learning on just one occasion would not be sufficient to result in a lifetime of stuttering. Imaging studies allow us to see the result of this learning by showing us 'what is happening where' in the brain when stuttering occurs and by showing when it is overcome by successful fluency techniques.

Imaging techniques, however, offer no explanation as to *how* or *why* these various neurophysiological processes are occurring or why they affect speaking. These images simply show us what is being activated and what is not. Now, this is a remarkable feat – of that there is no doubt – but it does not suggest an etiology. These results may simply reflect the result of years of stuttering on central nervous system functions rather than showing us anything about the cause of the stuttering: a frustrating example of the ancient chicken/egg conundrum. As Starkweather (1991: p. 386) reminded us:

> Even morphological differences, including those that have been observed in the central and peripheral speech mechanisms of stutterers, are just as likely to be results of the unusual patterns of social and communicative experience that

stutterers live through from an early age as they are to be a source of the disorder. Indeed the brain has been known for quite some years to develop in ways that reflect the individual's experience. This may help to explain why it is not just stutterers who are likely to have mixed cerebral dominance but also learning-disabled, deaf, articulation-disordered, and language-delayed children.

Imaging and activation studies are fairly clear cut and demand less inference than emotional/psychological and learning contributions, yet these also add to the processes that result in stuttering. Just as there are speech and motor control centres in the brain, so there are also cortical and sub-cortical areas and structures responsible for the internal and external manifestations of emotional arousal and response. These centres are also capable of influencing motor acts in both positive and negative ways. In the case of certain sub-cortical areas and structures it may well be the case that these are responsible for the aberrant activations and motor area hyperactivity reported by many imaging and activation studies.

Learning is an integral component of the syndrome of stuttering. Learning certainly does not exist in a neurophysiological void. We learn what we need to learn. We are 'told' what we need to learn through the evaluation of stimuli by areas of the brain concerned with emotional evaluation and cognitive understanding and evaluation. Often we remember things and really have no idea why we committed them to memory – perhaps they had no obvious cognitive value but they must have had an emotional value, at least at some time in our life. Memory is more complex than the discussion here but suffice it to say now that many of the cortical and (especially) sub-cortical areas responsible for our remembering are the same areas responsible for the emotional inputs that result in our internal and external manifestations of emotional arousal. So it would make sense that a component of the decision to store an experience in memory would be at least partially based on the emotional impact of that experience.

Reinforcement also influences what we remember. School grades and reactions from parents or significant others help goad us into studying harder (as does the satisfaction of learning and understanding for its own sake – if that is important to us). We remember best those things that gave us satisfaction, pleasure, happiness, contentment as well as pain, embarrassment, anxiety, or fear. We remember the positive so that we remember to repeat the circumstances that lead to it; we remember the negative so that we remember to try not to repeat the circumstances that lead to it. This is a very simplified explanation but it catches the essence of the basis of the process.

In order for us to pass data into long-term memory for much later, that information must first be stored and evaluated by our short-term memory. One structure critical for short-term memory and therefore for our long-term memory is the hippocampus. The hippocampus (so named because of its resemblance to a seahorse – although it always reminded me of a worm, thicker at one end, that was having difficulty negotiating a turn) is a sub-cortical structure that is considered a part of the limbic system – an area that we will discuss later. The hippocampus evaluates the incoming stimuli for importance and impact. Part of this process is assisted by the other structures of the limbic system that are responsible for all of our internal emotional states and for the external manifestations of those emotions. So how we respond emotionally to an experience helps determine whether we will remember it half an hour later (in the case, say, of the telephone number of the local video store) or whether we will remember it a year from now (as in the case of a wedding anniversary – the consequences of forgetting presumably being worse than having to look up the number of the video store again).

The structures of the limbic system that are responsible for our emotions have inputs from all the lobes of both hemispheres and send information back to sub-cortical and cortical structures and areas of those lobes. What this means is that the limbic structures evaluate and respond to all sensory data entering the central nervous system. In addition, the limbic system recalls and initiates emotional reactions and responses upward to the cortex for perception and incorporation into thought and behavioural responses. Recall that the hippocampus – responsible for both short- and long-term memory – is a part of this emotional system. If you remember a particularly embarrassing moment in your life, that memory is accompanied by memories of the feelings of embarrassment; if you remember a particularly joyous moment, those feelings are also an integral part of your memory. This is because the limbic system – through the hippocampus and other structures and areas responsible for long-term memory – is responding again to the memory of that incident.

The structures of this emotional system also have direct and indirect input into sub-cortical and cortical areas and structures responsible for the generation of language, speech and the interpretation of all other language output and input modalities. Many studies have documented that the limbic system can interfere with fluent speech as well as other voluntary motor acts. It is the contention of this manuscript that the aberrant activations and hyperactivity of motor areas identified by many imaging studies of stuttering are the result, to one degree or another, of input into other sub-cortical and cortical areas and structures by the limbic system.

Diagnostic implications

You might be asking yourself: 'Self, this is all well and good but what difference does it make?' The answer – as with most answers in response to a question stated in simple sentence form – is complex. Basically, though, the impact of consideration of the emotional/motor limbic system is important diagnostically because this information may well change your diagnostic protocols. The information, and yes, opinions and inferences, presented later on in this text will hopefully convince you that doing a stuttering frequency count and other 'standard', 'objective' measurements may not be the best source of information concerning the stuttering problem that your client is experiencing. You might also be asking: 'Why has he put those quotation marks around the words "standard" and "objective"?' Another good question: it is because recent reports suggest that it is a mistake to assume that you, as the listening clinician, know when a stuttering event has occurred. All frequency count measurements are based on the assumption that the clinician as listener is better able than the speaker who stutters in determining this decision. Just because something is counted does not suggest that it is a valid or objective method. What you count as a stuttering event might very well not be considered as such by the client.

Secondly, the limbic system emotional centres communicate with motor areas for speech and input of prosody into speech. It would be useful to determine before treatment how much attention will have to be paid to the underlying emotional reaction to stuttering that the client demonstrates (behavioural therapists have just closed the book at this point – but bear with me as so-called non-emotional, unanxious stuttering will also be addressed later). For instance, recent reports suggest that those clients who demonstrate an increased internal locus of control over their speech are those who improved the most and were expected to experience less reassertion of the stuttering behaviours. Diagnostically, then, the Locus of Control Scale could be a valuable tool in the determination of who will and who will not require the most treatment attention in terms of their internal emotional reactions to stuttering and who will be the most successful with the use of fluency enhancing techniques. It may also aid in predicting the success of long-term remedies for the stuttering.

Treatment implications

An appreciation of the underlying neurological basis of stuttering will have direct impact on the treatment recommended. As with any treatment consideration, the age of the client and the severity of the stuttering will be paramount considerations. This understanding of the neurology of the behaviour will be important in several ways. It will allow the therapist to identify the neurological targets of treatment techniques. For instance, instead of recommending that 'prosody' be targeted, one could state that the anterior area of Ross on the right hemisphere be the target of prosodic exercises to decrease the monotone associated with the use of delayed auditory feedback and the slowed, extended, but fluent speech that results from its use as a fluency enhancer. In other words, instead of using output as treatment targets one would be better able to conceptualize the origination points as targets.

Treatment bias is based on etiologic belief. If one believes that stuttering is best explained through learning theory it is doubtful that locus-of-control counselling techniques will constitute the majority of the treatment provided. However, if one is convinced by the information in this text, one will understand more about the contributions of learning *and* the emotional reactions to stuttering that are the basis of the development and maintenance of stuttering. One would hopefully then appreciate the how and why concerning the mutual importance of incorporating both counselling and learning techniques into therapy. Both have roots emanating from common neurological areas and structures. Treatment using both reinforces favourable speech outcomes.

What I have attempted to do in this manuscript is to present a unifying theory of stuttering: one that incorporates the perspectives of learning, emotion and neurology into a theoretical framework that can hopefully be used to better explain the acquisition and maintenance of stuttering behaviour. A theory should do more than explain; it should also generate treatments. Hopefully, this has been accomplished as well.

Chapter One
Neurophysiological review

If you think stuttering is complicated consider the act of speaking upon which stuttering is carried. In their book *Motor Speech Disorders,* Darley, Aronson and Brown (1975) estimated that fluent speech requires 140 000 neuromuscular events per second of speech. Consider, too, that these events must be programmed, co-ordinated, and performed flawlessly. It is a wonder that stuttering is not the norm and that we do not treat fluent speech as the disorder. These 140 000 events are the final result of input from a multitude of central and peripheral neurological sites into the muscles of the entire motor speech system.

It is the purpose of this chapter to present and review current neuro-physiological literature that delineates the locations and contributions of each of these cortical and sub-cortical areas and structures that collectively contribute to the final outcome of speech. Later in Chapter Two this information will describe the results of neuroimaging studies that show what is occurring within the central nervous system during fluent and stuttered speech.

Subcortical areas and structures

In the basement of both hemispheres lie those structures that have been collectively referred to as the limbic system. The word 'limbic' is derived from the Latin *limbus,* meaning ring or circle. Broca discovered this series of bilaterally represented structures that formed a ring around the inferior portions of the hemispheres and gave them this name. The human limbic system makes up what classical anatomists once referred to as the rhinen-cephalon or nosebrain. It was called this because these early anatomists believed that the primary responsibility of this area of the brain was the perception of the sense of smell. We now know that this ancient part of the central nervous system is the seat of both internal emotional states and the external manifestations of those internal states. But it is concerned with even more than that. The limbic system is the survival centre; it is from here that your body is thrust into the flight-or-fight mode. In the face of danger, emotional or physical, your body undergoes some serious changes. The senses are sharpened, blood is re-routed deeper into the body and adrenaline is released into the blood allowing faster reaction times and more strength. All of these and other responses by the limbic system set the body up to either stand and fight or to run. In the remote past, this flight-or-fight response was triggered in reaction to physical threats – the lion entering the cave, for instance; now this same set of responses is triggered if either physical or emotional threat is perceived. For instance, if we have to stand and give an oral presentation, our body reacts in much the same way to this circumstance as it would to facing an intruder in our home in the middle of the night. Our pulse and heartbeat increases, our stomach tightens (in response to the adrenaline released by the adrenal glands) and our palms sweat. It is our choice to either approach the podium or run from the room. In most cases we are able to control ourselves and approach the podium – even though we might fear it.

But what happens when we begin to speak to the multitude assembled to hear our lecture? Do we sound the same as when we are speaking privately with our friends? Is our rate of speech the same? Is our pitch the same? Is our intensity the same? Do we tend to 'mis-speak'? In other words, are we as natural sounding and fluent as when discussing what to have for lunch with friends? With practice, public speakers can sound natural and calm; but speakers new to oral presentations are usually nervous and stressed – and they sound that way. Why? How does a perceived threat to, say, our ego, affect the way that we speak? Look to the basements of your hemispheres for the answer. As will be illustrated below, limbic structures affect all aspects of the speech system. Our internal emotional states are reflected in our voice and in our fluency of speech production. Emotion is carried on the so-called suprasegmentals – stress, pause, pitch, intensity and the like. Emotion also affects fluency – witness the nervous speech of the novice public speaker, or the nervousness of the man proposing marriage, or the college student calling home for more money. Damage to cortical areas responsible for the input of suprasegmentals into speech results in a monotonous voice regardless of the emotionality of the message. This occurs because the limbic structures have lost the cortical transfer station located on the right frontal lobe in an area that mirrors the location of Broca's area on the left.

Historical review

Research into the etiology of emotion has a long and interesting history. In 1884, William James, the psychologist and brother of the novelist Henry James, put forth a theory of emotional perception based on his own introspective analysis when calling up emotional memories from his own experience. James believed that we feel emotions because of visceral changes that occur in response to stimuli. He thought that the visceral responses that we felt constituted the emotional state associated with the stimuli. In other words, he thought that we felt sadness *because* we cried, anger *because* we swung a fist, or fear *because* our knees were knocking. He did not believe that any visceral or body changes occurred in response to the emotion felt. Not long after James published his work, CG Lange (Arnold, 1968) theorized that emotion was essentially the result of vascular constriction in the viscera. These two theories so supported each other that they were grouped together and were thereafter referred to as the James–Lange theory of emotion.

In 1927, WB Cannon published his now famous rebuttal entitled *The James–Lange Theory of Emotion: a Critical Examination and an Alternative Theory*. In this, Cannon refuted the James–Lange theory with scientific evidence of the day. Cannon's work suggested that total separation of the viscera from the central nervous system does not impair emotional behaviour. He went on to show that the same visceral changes that James described as emotion occur in different emotional states and even in non-emotional states. Cannon demonstrated that the viscera are relatively insensitive structures due to poor sensory innervation. Further, Cannon considered that the viscera have too long a latency of central nervous system perception to be a source of emotional feeling.

In contrast to James and Lange, Cannon theorized that emotion was the product of the central nervous system. Essentially Cannon and then a colleague named Bard (1929), whose name became tied to Cannon's as Lange's was to James's, proposed that emotional experience was the result of thalamic functioning whereas emotional behaviour was attributed to the functioning of the hypothalamus.

The physiologist to whom modern research owes the most in terms of the investigation into emotional experience and functions, however, is JW Papez. In 1937, Papez published the landmark study, *A Proposed Mechanism of Emotion*. For the first time a number of brain structures were identified for individual and collective contribution to emotion. These were described by Papez as a 'circuit of emotion' (p. 289). Papez proposed that this circuit composed of the hypothalamus, cingulate gyrus and the hippocampus (has this term been held in your short-term memory?) and the interconnections between these structures comprised what Papez termed the 'anatomical seat of emotion' (p. 289). Sixty years of subsequent neurophysiological research has expanded this simple circuit of emotion into what is presently referred to as the limbic system of the human brain.

Current review

In addition to the commonly known characteristics of mammals (such as warm-bloodedness and live births) one may add the presence of common limbic structures (Isaacson, 1974). All mammals possess an amygdala, septum, hypothalamus and thalamus. It is in *homo sapiens*, however, that these and the other structures referred to previously 'culminate in development to allow humankind the wide range of emotional colouring, subtlety, and nuance characteristic of our species' (Livingston, 1978: p. 19).

The human limbic system makes up what classical anatomists once referred to as the *rhinencephalon* or 'nose-brain.' Prior to the work of Cannon, Bard and Papez, this portion of the brain was thought to be primarily concerned with olfaction. This ancient part of the brain was thought to be so concerned with the sense of smell that the area was relegated minimal responsibility for any higher-order functions (Isaacson, 1974).

According to Livingston (1978), one of the greatest advantages for humankind is our ability to deliver at birth an incompletely developed brain. Among the systems developing primarily after birth is the limbic system. The role of this system, then, could be shaped, according to Livingston, 'morphologically as well as functionally, in accordance with infantile and early childhood experiences' (p. 19). This simple observation has enormous meaning as the child develops into an adult.

> The attachment of the young to real or foster parents, to a varied and peculiar environment, and in many forms, to a culture, including in humans the facile initial acquisition of a language, is considered to represent an experimental link between limbic development and its capacity to attach values to biologically significant experiences. (Livingston, 1978: p. 19)

The importance of limbic development to the development for the brain as a whole has also been addressed. It is perhaps this single responsibility that best points to the crucial importance of limbic structures to brain function and to the developing child.

> This generalized laying down of memory stores is thought to be critically served or advantaged by limbic mechanisms (Livingston, 1978: p. 19).

Smythies (1968: p. 98) also credits the limbic system with 'executive control' and 'central co-ordinating' functions over the rest of the brain:

> It appears that the hippocampus, the amygdala, the septal nuclei, together with the 'limbic cortex', the hypothalamus, certain thalamic nuclei and the reticular formation may form the central co-ordinating and executive mechanism in the brain controlling such factors as memory formation, motivation, reinforcement, elaboration of emotions, [and] conditioned reflexes.

The limbic system, then, is certainly concerned with much more than olfaction or even the complexities of human emotion. It is also very involved in what is remembered, whether it is remembered in a positive or negative sense, and to what extent these memories and past associations influence present similar behaviours and coping strategies.

The limbic system, however, is not only involved with memory, associations, and emotion. It also influences vocalizations in primates and vocalizations and speech in man (Joseph, 1982; Jurgens, 1969; Kaada, 1951, 1967; Robinson, 1967). According to Robinson (1967), primate vocalizations resulting from sexual arousal, fear, anger, flight, or helplessness are primarily limbic and somatosensory based. Joseph (1982) states that 'in human infants the first vocalizations arise in response to somatosensory upheavals'. Hence, primate, including human, vocalizations arise at first in a context deeply embedded in limbic activity. Joseph continues by crediting virtually all human infant vocalizations to limbic influence:

> Because the limbic system monitors and responds to internal and external sensations (e.g., hunger, pain, etc.) with only minimal inhibitory regulation by the newborn's neocortex, most, if not all 'behaviour' is governed by brainstem and limbic concerns, including that of the first (and later) vocalizations. Hence, in response to hunger, the infant cries and to pleasure it gurgles and babbles. (p. 15)

These vocalizations become verbalizations over time. Limbic influences at this stage allow emotional expression to be conveyed through the suprasegmentals (Joseph, 1982).

Vocalization by the older child and adult is also limbically influenced. These types of limbically induced vocalizations involve the signal of danger, the cry of pain simultaneous with a reflexive withdrawal, or the grunt that accompanies heavy lifting or strenuous activity (Joseph, 1982).

Individuals with massive left-hemisphere damage who have lost expressive and receptive speech and language are reported by Geschwind (1968) to be able to sing, cry, swear, and, in some cases, pray. Joseph (1982) credits these abilities to the right (non-dominant) hemisphere, the orbital areas of the frontal lobes, and regions of the right temporal cortex. These areas, according to Kaada (1967) and Maclean (1954) are outgrowths of limbic nuclei that have maintained functional as well as cytoarchitectural similarities to the left-sided limbic lobe cortex.

We will see later in this review that several of the other cortical and subcortical areas and structures identified by more current researchers as possible contributors to stuttering are also considered to be evolutionary projections from limbic areas.

In addition to vocalizations and verbalizations in humans, Joseph (1982) credits limbic input as being responsible for the inflectional, suprasegmental aspects of speech through which additional nuance of meaning and emotionality is communicated. According to Joseph, these limbic suprasegmentals are fed to Broca's area, that 'final common pathway by which thought, emotion, and other impulses come to be organized as motoric articulations' (p. 22). The route by which this limbic influence may be communicated to Broca's area appears to be through bilateral subcortical and cortical areas and structures, especially via an anterior frontal area of the right hemisphere, the anterior area of Ross.

The limbic system, then, is involved with emotion, learning, memory, associations, and speech and language: all of which, of course, are involved with stuttering. To this point, this system has been referred to in general terms. The limbic system is made up of specific structures with individual intra- and interconnections, and functions. The following section addresses the anatomy, connections, and functions of these structures. Sorting through these interconnecting pathways can be a daunting task – as any graduate student in neurophysiology will attest. Hopefully the simplified diagrams that follow in Chapter Three will ease this task.

The amygdala

An axiom of our experience is the separate realities of our minds and bodies. The amygdala lies, functionally and anatomically, between these two poles, between the enormous thinking mantle that creates an objective mood of external reality, and the subjective inner reality of pain and fear, of surviving to mate and making sure that our offspring do also. The amygdala fits so well this paradoxical axis of human existence from biology to spirit that it has a tendency to achieve mythical status that goes beyond its true significance. One suspects that if the amygdala did not exist, it would have been invented as a metaphor for the connection of mind and body. (Halgren, 1992: p. 217)

The amygdala is located beneath the medial surface of the cerebral cortex in the pole of each temporal lobe (Isaacson, 1974; Guyton, 1976; Van Hoesen, 1995). Traditionally, as with the rest of the limbic system, the amygdala was considered to be primarily concerned with olfactory associations in humans and lower animals (Guyton, 1976). Its contributions, especially from its basolateral nuclei, have evolved in humans to include important roles in behaviour not associated with olfaction (Guyton, 1976). According to Guyton (1976: p. 765), in human beings:

The amygdala receives impulses from all portions of the limbic cortex, from the orbital surfaces for the frontal lobes, from the cingulate gyrus, and from the hippocampal gyrus. In turn, it transmits signals (a) back into these same cortical areas, (b) into the hippocampus, (c) into the septum, (d) into the thalamus, and (e) especially into the hypothalamus.

In addition, these paired temporal lobe structures also communicate with one another via the inferior commissure (Smythies, 1966).

Electrical stimulation studies of various aspects of the amygdala have yielded a wide range of somatomotor reactions, visceral reactions and behavioural reactions. Smythies (1966) reports that such stimulation of the lateral division of the amygdaloid nucleus results in movements of the eyes, head, face and jaw. These movements may either be clonic or tonic. He also reports results of arrest of spontaneous movements in experimental animals (species not reported). The amygdala has direct communication with the thalamus and, through it, to other structures of the basal ganglia, all of which communicate with the prefrontal motor areas, the supplementary motor areas and the primary motor areas of the brain (Guyton, 1976).

Since the seventies, however, new information has emerged that expands on the amygdala–basal ganglia links. It is now known that these connections are not through the thalamus exclusively. Amaral (1993) reported that the amygdala–striatum projections constitute one of the greatest outputs, if not *the* greatest output, of the amygdala. These efferents link the amygdala with the putamen, the caudate nucleus and even with the substantia nigra.

All of these areas have been implicated by current neuroimaging studies as being activated during stuttering in the researchers' subjects who stuttered. This will be explored in the following chapters. For now, though, keep the amygdala–basal ganglia connectors in mind as you read.

Kaada (1951), in reporting the results of an extensive study involving electrical stimulation of the amygdala in primates, cats, dogs and humans, reported complete respiratory arrest in the expiratory cycle. Arrest was more pronounced with stimulation of the medial aspect of the monkey's amygdala. This arrest could only be held for 25 to 35 seconds, after which physiological escape occurred and the monkeys breathed normally. Hypothesizing that he could have inadvertently stimulated other areas, he repeated the procedure and obtained the same results. Kaada (1951) reported that similar results were obtained from the same procedure using cats and dogs. In addition to replicating the results obtained from monkeys by using cats as subjects, Kaada was able to produce chewing movements with the jaws of the experimental animals.

Stimulation and ablation studies have reported results ranging from flight, what Kaada (1972) reports as a fear reaction, to defence and then attack behaviour in cats. Bard (1961) reports that when bilateral removal of the amygdala is performed on the macaque monkey, an experimental animal known for its 'normally aggressive and intractable behaviour' (p. 1191), it abolishes or significantly reduces this primate's normal aggressiveness and its reactions to fear. Additional evidence of the impact on behaviour of the bilateral removal of the amygdala is shown by the effect of the procedure upon the wild Norway rat, a 'savage and untameable creature' (Bard, 1961: p. 1191). Following surgery, the rats were 'rendered gentle and innocuous' (p. 1191). In addition, depending on the sites, electrical stimulation of the amygdala can also produce rage, escape, pain, or pleasure (Guyton, 1976).

The role of the amygdala, however, is not even limited to these widely diverse responses as it also has connections with the pituitary adrenal stress mechanism (Smythies, 1966). These findings are not surprising as, in humans, electrical stimulation of deep structures of the amygdala most often produces the very unpleasant sensation of uncontrollable fear (Gloor, 1972; Mullan and Penfield, 1959; Jasper and Rasmussen, 1958; Strauss, Risser and Jones, 1982). Fear results in stress and in the pituitary's reaction with adrenocorticotropic hormone (ACTH) and adrenaline production and secretion.

What the amygdala tells the rest of the brain, through the thalamus and hypothalamus, is directly related to an individual's perception of the environment, including memory, associations, and learning. Researchers have determined that the amygdala either excites or inhibits a specific set of neurones in the hypothalamus (Gloor, 1978: pp. 203–4). Gloor proposes that 'the amygdala either "activates" or "inhibits" some functions which are controlled by the hypothalamus, and that the "decision" to do one or the other depends upon the "content" of the message received (by the amygdala) from the neo-cortex'. Gloor summarizes his theory of amygdaloid functioning as the structure that will 'provide what may be called the appropriate "affective bias" or perhaps more anthropomorphically, the appropriate "mood" which is normally evoked by a constellation of environmental stimuli to which the animal is exposed' (p. 204). He further states that in such a schema, learning, not inborn mechanisms, must play the most crucial role: 'It is therefore likely that the most common, the most frequently recurrent perceptual constellations which have acquired definite affective connotations in the past, must be most effective in determining the affective response mediated by the amygdala' (p. 205).

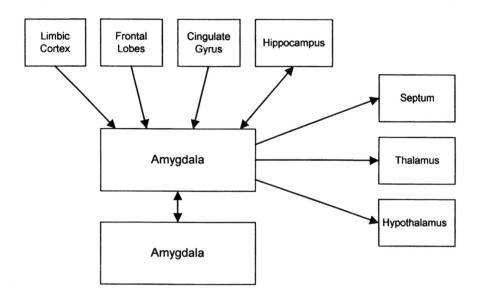

Figure 1.1: Connections to the amygdala.

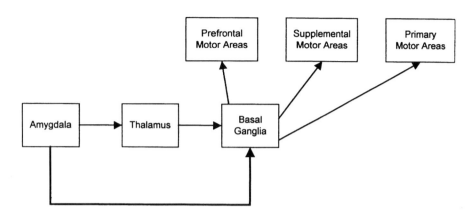

Figure 1.2: Amygdala thalamic projections – heavy line indicates greatest output.

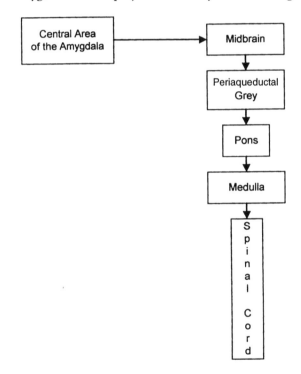

Figure 1.3: Amygdala–brainstem connections.

This 'affective response' or 'emotional' biasing by the amygdala also extends into the realm of social interaction. Gloor reports that monkeys who had their amygdalas ablated or removed appeared to lose appropriate pre-learned social behaviours within their social group. Such monkeys, when released back into their communal cages preferred to stay back from the group, to remove themselves from the necessity of social interaction with which they had been unable to cope. Wild monkeys that

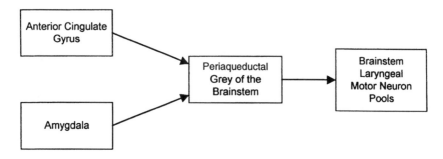

Figure 1.4: Amygdala connections with PAG.

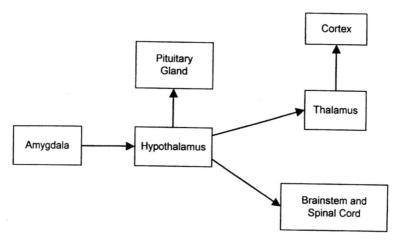

Figure 1.5: Major pathways from the hypothalamus.

had undergone the same procedure but were released back in to the wild 'ran away from their former companions and hid in inaccessible caves or other lonely outposts' (p. 207). The amygdala, then, either directly or indirectly influences behaviour related to appropriate social interaction. The amygdala may influence appropriateness of social behaviour in accordance with the individual's perception of the environment, memory stores, associations and learning.

In addition to the above connections with other subcortical structures and areas the amygdala also has direct and profuse connections with the midbrain, brainstem and even the spinal cord (Amaral et al., 1993). Fibres from the central areas of the amygdala travel into and through the midbrain where they connect with the periaqueductal grey, the pons and the medulla. Below the medulla, some continue down into the spinal cord.

In their travels through the structures of the brainstem, the amygdala fibres innervate a number of areas that affect speech performance. For instance, one such area is the dorsal motor nucleus for the vagus nerve.

The vagus gives rise to the superior and recurrent laryngeal nerves that are responsible for vocal fold adduction, abduction and pitch change. In addition, the amygdala connects with the periaqueductal grey of the midbrain. This area acts as a relay station between the cortex and the vagal motor nucleus and the nerves responsible for the above laryngeal actions. The amygdala, then, has ample input into motor control of the larynx.

This input is via direct brainstem innervation of the vagus cranial nerve as well as through the connections between the amygdala and the basal ganglia. Amaral (1993) demonstrated that these connections between the amygdala and the structures of the basal ganglia constitute the largest output collection of fibres from the amygdala. These fibres join the amygdala with the ventral and medial portions of the caudate nucleus, the putamen, and the nucleus accumbens in the ventral area of the striatum as well as the substantia nigra. The structures of the basal ganglia or striatum are also integral parts of the extrapyramidal system. This, the second major motor system in the brain, is one of the etiological areas for the motor and speech deficits associated with Parkinson's disease.

Until recently there has been little anatomical evidence for direct connections between the amygdala and the hippocampus. Due to the strength of olfactory and emotional memory such links were assumed. We now know that such links exist – just as hypothesized (Amaral, 1993). These links can only be demonstrated in primates; none has been found (yet) in cats, rats, or dogs. They are probably there in dogs though. The links from the hippocampus to the amygdala are not as profuse, probably because they are not as crucial. What would be crucial to the laying in of emotional memory would be the input from the amygdala to the hippocampus, not the opposite. However, motor responses to learned behaviour are very dependent upon both short-term and long-term memory and inputs from these memory areas to the basal ganglia.

Although probably not central to the thesis of this text, but interesting nonetheless, is the fact that the amygdala receives a great deal of visual input. What we see is available for the amygdala – and through it the rest of the limbic system – to evaluate, to attach emotionality to it. This certainly makes sense as anyone moved by a picture, sunset, or his or her child's face will attest. Speaking of faces – we now also know that the amygdala is a part of the facial recognition complex. Classically, areas of the right hemisphere have received the most credit for our ability to recognize faces (a much more complicated skill than would 'meet the eye'). A group of neurones in the amygdala only responds to visual input of faces (Rolls, 1993).

The contribution of the amygdala in this area is to help identify the face so that emotional meaning can be assigned to it and appropriate social responses can be elicited from the emotional memory stores or can be assigned to emotional memory stores for future evocation. As will be remembered from above (how's that hippocampus of yours doing?)

ablation studies implicate the amygdala in elicitation of appropriate social responses. It would therefore be important for the amygdala to be able to recognize and respond to the faces that we encounter.

Assigning emotional responses to what we hear would also be important to our emotional responsiveness. The amygdala therefore has extensive connections with the auditory cortex and the auditory association areas of the cortex. These connections are easy for the amygdala since its location in the medial temporal lobes gives easy and direct access to these areas (Van Hoesen, 1995). Interestingly, though, there are more connections with the visual cortices than the auditory areas (Amaral, 1993).

With all of these connections to and from the cortex, can connections with the frontal lobes, insula and anterior cingulate gyrus be far behind? Obviously, the answer is no. The amygdala has profuse connections with these cortices as well. There are many more connections with the anterior portions of all these areas than with medial or posterior portions. The denseness falls off fairly dramatically the further posteriorly one follows these fibres in all of the above areas. Fibres connect the amygdala with the agranular insular cortex, the lateral orbital cortex, the medial orbital cortex and the medial wall of the frontal lobe (Amaral, 1993). All of these areas are densely innervated by the amygdala. Different amygdaloid nuclei connect with different areas of these cortices. Many of these same areas are activated during stuttering.

Both the anterior cingulate gyrus (Jurgens and Von Cremon, 1982) and the amygdala have extensive connections with the periaqueductal grey (PAG) of the midbrain (Kapp, Whalen, Supple, and Pascoe, 1993). The PAG has recently been proposed as a transfer station through which emotional arousal is communicated into motor speech (Denny and Smith, 1997). In this model the PAG is seen as a co-ordinator of limbic emotional responses and motor activity, including speech. Stimulation of the PAG 'produces strongly and consistently patterned motor responses that effectively take over muscles of the chest wall, larynx and face' (p. 129). In their model, Denny and Smith (1997) posit respiration and laryngeal control abnormalities as being the crux of stuttering behaviour. Due to contributions of the PAG to both these areas in speech, Denny and Smith state:

> The potential importance of the PAG for stuttering is that, like the metabolic respiratory controller, it can influence the entire speech musculature. Second, it is essential for the organization of emotional expression . . . The possibility that the PAG may contribute disruptive inputs into motoneurone pools that originate from the brainstem circuitry in disordered speakers remains to be studied. (p. 130)

It is , of course, proposed here that limbic inputs from the amygdala and the anterior cingulate gyrus of the cortex produce the PAG activations that do, in fact, contribute to stuttering. Denny and Smith summarize their theory concerning respiration, laryngeal functioning and stuttering in the following:

During normal speech, there is a reduction of inputs into motoneurone pools that originate from the brainstem circuitry responsible for metabolic (life support) breathing and/or the PAG, which is active for emotional vocalization. Respiratory and laryngeal function is taken over and managed primarily by the speech controller. In contrast, in individuals who stutter, the metabolic and emotional-vocal centres, for a variety of reasons, may compete with the speech control system. The interaction and competition of these control systems may be a source of instability in speech motor control for individuals who stutter. (p. 130)

Jurgens (1994) and Jurgens and Zwirer (1997) support Denny and Smith's contentions that the PAG is an emotional relay centre and that there is an additional input site for motor speech that involves instructions for speech. These researchers found that pharmacological blocking of the PAG in primate subjects abolished vocalization controlled by the cingulate gyrus and hypothalamus but not vocalization initiated by the neocortex. Jurgens and Zwirer consider these results to support the existence of two separate vocal fold control paths at the midbrain PAG level. One of these pathways is limbic and is responsible for emotional utterances; the other originates from the cortex and is responsible for learned patterns of vocal-ization. The PAG is viewed in this model – much as in the model of Denny and Smith – as a crucial relay station for the limbic but not the cortically based vocalizations.

This work of Jurgens and Zwirer supports both the Denny and Smith model as well as the position of this text: the PAG represents yet another major input source of disruptive limbically based emotional learning into speech production. Combining both the Denny and Smith and the limbic model under presentation here a near perfect fit is established. Denny and Smith postulated two control systems for speech, one a speech controller and the other an emotionally based speech disrupter that was represented as the PAG. The limbic model presents the PAG as one of several input areas of disruptive limbically based inputs into speech. Denny and Smith maintain that input from the speech controller is disrupted by competi-tion with the emotional inputs from the PAG. The Denny and Smith model stops at the PAG. The limbic model under presentation here takes the origination to the sources of inputs into the PAG that are then fed into speech at that point. Those ultimate sources include the amygdala, hypothalamus, anterior cingulate gyrus and other areas to be discussed.

So, the amygdala has all of these (mostly) reciprocal connections with sensory areas of the cortex, with important sub-cortical motor areas, with the midbrain, brainstem and cranial nerve nuclei located there, as well as transfer stations for innervation of the larynx, and even to the spinal cord. In addition to all this, the amygdala has direct connections with the hypothalamus and hippocampus and through these structures to the rest of the limbic areas (neurophysiology would be easier if we only studied what was not connected to something else). So (again) this little almond shaped structure (that's where it got the name amygdala) sends and receives information to all areas involved in sensation, movement, and emotional response and memory formation and storage. It really is well located, anatomically and functionally, to act as a bridge between what we feel and how that feeling is remembered as well as what effects that emotion or emotional memory has on our behaviour and movements. We will return to the amygdala as well as other topics in this chapter when we discuss learning, memory, movement, and the effect of sub-cortical input on behaviour.

The hypothalamus

The hypothalamus 'in all vertebrates makes up the floor of the third ventricle' (Bard, 1961: p. 118). It appears smaller in lower animals than in more highly evolved mammals. It is closely associated with the medial forebrain bundle, which, according to Bard, 'arises in the ventromedial centres of the cerebral hemisphere' (p. 1182). These centres include the olfactory bulb and peduncle, the anterior perforated substance, the septum, the paraolfactory region, and the amygdaloid nucleus. The fibres of this tract run into and through the thalamus.

The question of what connects the hypothalamus with brain areas and structures outside of the limbic system per se is controversial due to the diffuseness, fineness and, for the most part, unmyelinated structure of its connections, all of which make delineation or staining difficult (Isaacson, 1974). However, evidence drawn from studies showing influences on the hypothalamus and effects on visceral, physiological and muscular reaction due to hypothalamic stimulation demonstrates there are afferent and efferent connections between the hypothalamus and other distinct aspects of the central nervous system (Bard, 1961).

As discussed earlier, there are direct connections between the amygdala and the hypothalamus. The amygdala is thought to exert either an inhibitory or facilitatory control over hypothalamic activity. The connections are reciprocal (Egger, 1972). The pathways are via the stria terminalis and the ventral amygdalofugal system (Egger, 1972). In addition to the direct pathways between the amygdala and hypothalamus, there are indirect pathways between them involving structures outside the limbic system. Egger informs us that 'in cats there may be a pathway from the amygdala to the hippocampus via the pyriform cortex and then to the hypothalamus via the fornix' (p. 32). According to Nauta (1962), in the monkey there is a pathway from the amygdala to the dorsomedial nucleus of the thalamus to the orbitofrontal cortex, and from there to the hypothalamus.

Of great interest is the evidence that there are direct projections from the pre-motor cortex, area 6, and from the posterior orbital cortex, area 13, which terminate in the ventromedial aspect of the hypothalamic nuclei (Clark, 1950). Wiesendanger (1981) reports that Fulton saw area 6 as synonymous with what he termed 'the premotor area'. According to cortical stimulation studies, area 6B controls facial expression, facial movements, mastication, and swallowing (Wiesendanger, 1981). Thalamic projections increase in number phylogenetically; therefore, humans have the greatest number of thalamic projections to this area. Area 6 is one of the cortical areas inappropriately activated during stuttered speech (Fox et al., 1996).

This premotor area has bilateral connections with what Penfield (1950) termed the 'supplementary motor area' (SMA). Vocalization is the most common result of electrical stimulation of the SMA of the left side. Other motor responses in human subjects include turning of the head and eyes to the side opposite the stimulation (Wiesendanger, 1981). Input to the SMA is predominantly from somatosensory signals, whereas the premotor cortex is specialized for visually guided movements. In the present context, area 6 presents a bridge from the amygdala to the SMA via the hypothalamus and thalamus.

Speech is a sensorimotor act, a fact on which Zimmerman (1980a, 1980b, 1980c) founded his model of stuttering. Zimmerman theorized that stuttering was the result of violated parameters of acceptable articulatory movements. The SMA and its rich connections with the somatosensory areas may be the central modulator in Zimmerman's model. As Wiesendanger (1981) reminds us: 'It is well to remember that one of the most prominent effects of SMA stimulation in man is vocalization or arrest of speech, an observation that led Penfield and Jasper to consider the SMA as a third speech centre' (p. 1135). If so, it would be the case that the modulation is disrupted by an inappropriate Area 6 activation due to limbic input via the amygdala and hypothalamus.

Pathways from the hypothalamus fall, according to Bard (1961), into three main groups. One courses to the thalamus and from that structure to the cortex; the second courses to the brain stem and spinal cord; the last runs to the pituitary gland. According to Gatz (1970), 'Conduction pathways between the hypothalamus and the cortex are diverse and in some cases circuitous' (p. 100). The major afferent connection of the hypothalamus is the fornix, a tract that ends in the mammillary nuclei. The efferent connection of these nuclei is the mammillothalamic tract, which directly connects with the anterior nucleus of the thalamus. The anterior thalamic nucleus connects with the cingulate gyrus, and the thalamus has direct connections with the neocortex. As you will see, the anterior portions of the cingulate gyrus and the thalamus make important contributions to speech. Of particular interest to this study is the fact that stimulation of the hypothalamus, as well as areas of the anterior limbic area (Kaada, 1951), can result in 'every known type of neurogenic effect in the cardiovascular system, including increased arterial pressure [and] increased heart rate' (Guyton, 1976: p. 760). Additionally, the hypothalamic input to the pituitary gland and its influences in the release of ACTH hormone, so closely linked with the subjective feeling of anxiety (Bard, 1961), as well as the pituitary's control of the adrenals and their hormonal output (Guyton, 1976; Smythies, 1966; Bard, 1961) are of significance in terms of the cyclic pattern of perception, anxiety, tension, and their roles in dysfluency. According to Bard (1961) hypothalamic output is dependent on the degree of emotional arousal: 'Without doubt the most marked and most general sympathetic discharges occur under conditions designated by Cannon as emergency states. These include states of strong emotion such as fear and anger' (p. 1188).

Additionally, stimulation of the hypothalamus results in activation of the motor cortex and an increase of pyramidal discharges. According to Gellhorn and Loofborrow (1963) this causes 'further intensification of these movements' (p. 76) initiated by the motor cortex and can result in tonic blocks of muscle movement. Taken collectively, the effects of motor acts by stimulation of the hypothalamus seem to mirror the clonic/tonic speech characteristics of stuttering as well as accompanying emotional reactions of anxiety and fear.

Another of the myriad functions of this extraordinary structure appears to involve anger, and in certain circumstances, true and 'sham' rage. Stimulation of the perifornical nucleus of the hypothalamus in cats and monkeys results in the animal assuming a defensive posture, extending its claws, hissing, spitting or growling, piloerection, and widening its eyes. The slightest provocation will result in an attack of extreme savageness (Guyton, 1976; Bard, 1961). As with many other hypothalamic functions, this savageness appears to be mediated in intact animals by the influence of the amygdaloid input to the ventromedial aspect of the hypothalamus. Localized destruction of these nuclei also results in previously docile, gentle cats becoming savage (Wheatley, 1944; Egger and Flynn, 1963. This would support the theory that the amygdala exerts influence via the hypothalamus and other structures in the setting of affective bias or 'mood' within individuals and their responses to the environment.

MacLean (1970) views the hypothalamus as playing a fundamental role in the integration of emotional expression via viscerosomatic behaviour. MacLean suggests that it is through the hypothalamus that many of the visceral reactions associated with emotions are generated.

Another interesting aspect of hypothalamic activity involves its role in learning and motivation. Smythies (1966) reports that partial ablation of the hypothalamus and the reticular formation resulted in the abolishment of an alimentary conditioned response, which left the unconditioned response intact. In other words, food will elicit salivation but the bell will not. He further reports that lesions in the area of the mammillary bodies result in interference with the acquisition of a conditioned aversive response (Smythies, 1966). Roberts, Steinberg, and Means (1976) and Lindsley (1970) report a motivational function of the hypothalamus. Stimulation of hypothalamic centres involving emotionally based and motivating behaviours such as mating, attacking, defensive eating, and grooming, resulted in those responses relevant to goals being elicited only in the presence of the goal objects. If the goal objects are not present, behaviour related to them (such as eating, drinking, grooming, or attacking) did not occur. Therefore, the hypothalamus-amygdala-hippocampus interface forms one of the bases of conditioned learning. These areas may be the foundation for the emotional and motor learning that is evidenced as stuttering.

As may be seen from this review, the hypothalamus is an exceedingly complex and powerful structure involved with vegetative functioning, emotional and motor responses, motivation and learning. Its extensive reciprocal communication with the amygdala, the premotor cortex, the SMA, the posterior orbital cortex, the frontal cortex, the pituitary and other structures comprising the limbic system, involves the hypothalamus with emotional perception and a wide variety of behavioural and visceral emotionally based responses.

The hippocampus

As with most other limbic structures, until recently the hippocampus, or 'archipallium' as it has been known, was accorded olfactory functions. However, according to Bard (1961), Guyton (1976), Smythies (1970) and Isaacson (1974), olfaction is definitely not one of the hippocampus's primary functions and Bard (1961) posits that the hippocampus has no relation to olfaction at all, as do current authors (Nolte, 1993).

The hippocampus has extensive connections with all parts of the limbic system, especially with the amygdala, the hippocampal gyrus, and the hypothalamus (Guyton, 1976). Smythies (1970) and Nolte (1993) report the following afferent connections to the hippocampus:

1. A pathway from the adjacent entorhinal area (hippocampal gyrus) that distributes via the alvear and perforant paths of Cajal to the dendrites of the pyramidal cells. This provides a pathway for impulses from the temporal lobe. There are extensive connections to the hippocampus from all regions of the temporal neocortex.
2. A pathway from the reticular formation running via the septum and fornix. The septal path to the hippocampus offers a means for activity ascending from the brainstem to reach the hippocampus.
3. Electrical studies in humans indicate the presence of a path from the thalamic reticular formation.
4. A two-way connection with the hippocampus of the opposite side via the hippocampal commissure.
5. A diffuse inflow from the limbic midbrain area via the subthalamic region. This may run via the septum in part.
6. The cingulum from the cingulate gyrus and the medial forebrain bundle (pp. 27–8).

They report the following main efferent connections:

1. A major pathway that runs via the fornix to the septal region, the preoptic area, much of the hypothalamus, the limbic zone of the midbrain reticular formation, dorsomedial and intralaminar thalamic nuclei and the mammillary bodies (and then to the Papez circuit).
2. An important pathway to the entorhinal area and thereby relay to the rest of the temporal lobe.
3. A direct route to the reticular formation via the subthalamic area.
4. There are diffuse two-way connections with the ipsilateral amygdala (pp. 28–9).

According to Smythies (1968), the hippocampus receives information about the state of the environment in a coded and analysed form. This information is then fed around the circuits of the limbic system 'in the form of an internal representation of the external world' (p. 88). At the same time, input from the amygdala is feeding data concerning visceral events into the same circuits (Smythies, 1968). Smythies suggests that the time relationship between these two inputs may be the foundation of conditioned reflex formation.

Thus the packet of schemata 'A' (such as the sound of a bell) circulated from the hippocampus at the same time or shortly before a packet of schemata 'B' originating from the amygdala indicating 'food in stomach,' then 'A' will be 'strengthened,' will remain in the programme and be laid down in the permanent memory store. If there is no 'B' it would simply die out and be lost. The actual centre computing these relationships may be the reticular formation on which both circuits impinge. The reticular formation is necessary for retention of recent memories (p. 88).

The author indicates that this experimental record is fed to the midbrain reticular formation and then to the thalamic reticular formation 'as a programme for motor behaviour and to the hypothalamus as a correlated programme for the visceral concomitants for behaviour ("emotion")' (Smythies, 1968, p. 88).

According to Guyton (1976), stimulation of unspecified parts of the hippocampus can result in tonic or clonic movements of the human body. However, Kaada's (1951) extensive investigation of electrical stimulation of various limbic structures consistently reported no motor responses from the hippocampus of dogs, cats, or humans. Authors agree that stimulation of the hippocampus in conscious individuals results in their temporarily losing contact with their environments and, more specifically, as reported by Guyton (1976), with any individual to whom they are speaking. Guyton attributes this phenomenon to the role of the hippocampus in determining a person's attention. This appears to be a very reasonable explanation since the hippocampus has two-way connections with the reticular formation. Additionally, there are probably reciprocal connections between the hippocampus and hypothalamus (Isaacson, 1974). This reciprocity is included in Arnold's 'action circuit' (1970, p. 270). According to Arnold, when

> Something is appraised as 'good for a particular action,' relays from the limbic cortex seem to run to the hippocampus and connect via the fornix, hypothalamus, midbrain, and cerebellum with the anterior ventral thalamic nuclei and the premotor and motor cortex. (1970: p. 270)

Arnold continues by stating that the appraisal part of this action circuit is mediated within the appropriate limbic structures, but that the 'felt tendency to move toward or away from something is mediated by the premotor cortex' (p. 270). This action circuit results in 'each appraisal (producing) a felt tendency to action which either leads directly to appropriate behaviour or is modified by subsequent appraisals and subsequent action tendencies, all mediated via the action circuit connecting with the frontal lobe' (Arnold, 1970, p. 271).

Besides the part played by the hippocampus as a part of various limbic circuits, it appears to have a role in memory functioning. Hippocampal lesions in humans most often result in anterograde amnesia, in which all prior memories are intact but the laying down of new memories after the trauma is severely inhibited (Guyton, 1976; Smythies, 1970; Isaacson, 1974). This is especially true for learning verbal information. According to Guyton (1976), this is probably due to the particular responsibility of the temporal lobes for this mode of communication. This type of lesion, however, has no effect on the individual's level of 'attention, concentration, reasoning ability, intelligence, vocabulary, or professional skills' (Smythies, 1970: p. 64).

In terms of limbic involvement, Guyton views the role of the hippocampus as providing 'a channel through which different incoming sensory signals can excite appropriate limbic reactions' (p. 765). He bases this observation on the fact that 'any type of sensory experience causes instantaneous activation of different parts of the hippocampus and the hippocampus in turn distributes many outgoing signals to the hypothalamus and other parts of the limbic system through the fornix' (p. 765).

Thus, the hippocampus may act as a limbic switching station directing information to various limbic structures and from this system to other distant brain areas via the hypothalamus, thalamus and amygdala.

The septum and septal area

All parts of the septum receive 'massive input from a wide variety of limbic regions as well as the hypothalamus' (Isaacson, 1974: p. 45). In human beings, the septal area is 'the most medial portion of the frontal lobe' (Smythies, 1970: p. 33).

The septal area has reciprocal connections with the hippocampus, amygdala, hypothalamus and reticular formation (Smythies, 1970; Isaacson, 1974). In addition, there are two pathways with septal connections, 'the stria terminalis to the reticular formation . . . and to the amygdala via the diagonal band of Broca. It also connects directly with the anterior, lateral reticular, dorsomedial, and other thalamic nuclei, and cingulate gyrus' (Smythies, 1970, pp. 33–4).

Due to its important role in arousal of the hippocampus, the septum has been hypothesized to be the most rostral portion of the reticular activating system. A septal lesion will block theta rhythm in the hippocampus, and stimulation of a patent septum will cause large potentials in the hippocampus (Smythies, 1970).

Lesions of the septum in non-primates result in an increase in attack behaviour and aggressiveness immediately after surgery (Isaacson, 1974). This savageness lessens over time and can be shortened further with daily handling of the animal, while hypothalamic lesions result in long-lasting hyper emotionality. The savageness after a septal lesion, according to Isaacson, is seen only in non-primates, although Smythies (1970) presents contradictory results with human subjects.

Reports of septal damage in humans show that coma, similar to that from a lesion of the midbrain portion of the reticular formation, is common. Septal tumours of the pellucidum in humans resulted in early symptoms similar to the septal syndrome in lesioned rats; that is, emotional irritability and aggressive outbursts and emotional lability (Smythies, 1970). Electrical stimulation of the septum also results in changes in blood pressure, respiratory rate and digestion (McKeough, 1982).

The septum appears to exert great influence over, and to have close functional ties with, the hippocampus in terms of arousal and inhibition of the hippocampus and the hippocampal role in emotionality (Smythies, 1970). The inhibitory aspect of septum involvement is evidenced by 'increases [in] emotionality when it is defined in terms of gross observations of the animal' (Hammond, 1970) when the septum has been surgically removed.

These intraconnections and interconnections of the limbic system suggest that one responsibility of the system as a whole is to maintain an organismic homeostasis that has been disrupted due to internally or externally generated stimuli. As Smythies (1968) has suggested, one role of the hippocampus is to feed 'an internal representation of the external world' (p. 88) around the limbic circuits and then to the rest of the appropriate far-brain sites for internal and behavioural response. It follows then that another aspect of hippocampal functioning, after arousal by the septum, would be to feed to these same limbic circuits internally generated responses to these stimuli.

The cingulate gyrus

Surrounding the corpus callosum on the medial aspect of the cerebrum is the cingulate gyrus. The cingulate gyrus receives fibres from the anterior thalamic nuclei. Considered an important portion of the limbic system, the anterior thalamic nuclei have profuse connections with the limbic system (Gatz, 1970). The cingulate gyrus also has 'direct connections with the hippocampus and with all other limbic areas' (Guyton, 1976: p. 766).

A variety of findings applicable to this investigation have been reported in research using electrical stimulation of various regions of the cingulate gyrus in primates but especially stimulation of points within the anterior portion. Although Smythies (1970) does not give stereotaxic descriptions of these stimulations, he reports general observations of the results of electrical stimulation. Stimulation of points within the anterior cingulate gyrus (ACG) yielded an arrest of respiration during exhalation. Other areas of stimulation resulted in an arrest of all spontaneous movement initiated by the primary motor area. When area four was activated simultaneously with the ACG, movements were 'inhibited, augmented, or first one then the other' (p.96), resulting in clonic motor movements. Smythies, however, reports the most common result of ACG stimulation is inhibition of ongoing motor activity.

Smythies (1970) considers the ACG to be a sensorimotor vagal area since many effects caused by stimulation of the ACG can also be obtained by stimulating the central, cut end of the vagus. In addition, a pathway has been identified that runs from the vagal nuclei via the hypothalamus and septal area of the ACG. Smythies also reported that tonic and clonic motor responses have been obtained from stimulation of the ACG. These movements occur even when the motor areas of both hemispheres have been extirpated. These movements, in the absence of the bilateral motor cortexes, point up the relative independence of movements associated with emotional reactions as opposed to movements initiated by the primary motor cortex.

Particularly relevant to this investigation are the observations that stimulation of the ACG can also result in vocalizations (Jurgens and Von Cremon, 1982; Jurgens and Muller-Preuss, 1977) and licking and chewing movements (Smythies, 1970). Kaada (1951), Showers and Crosby (1958) and Robinson (1967) all obtained vocalization by stimulating the ACG of the rhesus monkey. In a review of their results of vocalization following stimulation of the ACG, Jurgens and Von Cremon (1982) considered these vocalizations to be independent of 'stimulational-induced motivational changes' (p. 234), such as vocalization in response to sexual or gustatory stimulation. Instead, they view the ACG as critical to volitional initiation of vocalization. In support of this position they point out: 'neuroanatomical studies . . . have shown that there is a pathway running from the ACG to the laryngeal motor-neurones with only one synapse in the area of the periaqueductal grey' (p. 234). Additionally, 'there are direct projections from the ACG to almost all other brain areas yielding vocalization when electrically stimulated' (p. 235). Finally, single-unit recording techniques have shown that

> there are a number of neurones in the anterior cingulate cortex of the monkey that change their activity a few hundred milliseconds prior to each vocalization uttered in a vocal conditioning situation; these neurones do not react however to other conditioned oral movements like biting or licking. (p. 235)

Behavioural changes have also been observed following stimulation of the ACG. Botez and Barbeau (1971) report that stimulation of the ACG resulting in vocalization in primates is 'always associated with emotional expressions such as opening the eyes or raising the frontalis muscle' (p. 301).

Studies of human cingulate lesions *in vivo* are rare due to the high mortality rate among individuals with trauma to the cingulate gyrus and adjacent brain areas (Jurgens and Von Cremon, 1982). Prior to succumbing to their injuries, however, the most common result of cingulate damage is mutism. Although these patients died before having regained speech abilities, Jurgens and Von Cremon hypothesized, based on animal studies, that the result of such trauma on human speech would impair volitional control of emotional utterances.

Jurgens and Von Cremon (1982) cited a rare and unusual case in which the patient survived cingulate lesions. They reported that, in March 1977, a patient was transferred to the Max Planck Institute in Munich, Germany and was seen, for the first time, by two physician-researchers. The patient's history is detailed.

On Christmas Eve, 1975, the 41-year-old right-handed man suddenly lost consciousness. Diagnostic evaluations revealed blockage of both anterior cerebral arteries. For six weeks the patient was mute. By February the patient was able to respond non-verbally to verbal commands given by the physicians. He made no effort to speak, despite the evaluation that his tongue and other articulators were functioning normally and that he could swallow with ease. Speech, in the form of whispering, returned by March of 1976. Although he was able to imitate long sentences, he would initiate vocalization only when prodded by his physician; otherwise, he would remain silent.

A computed tomography scan revealed a bilateral infarction in the area of both anterior cerebral arteries. Detailed examination of the scan revealed that the lesion had invaded the ACG bilaterally as well as the SMA unilaterally, the medial orbital cortex bilaterally, and the most rostral portion of the striatum. Jurgens and Von Cremon posited that their patient's speech difficulty was not the result of damage or interruption of the cortical output from the classical motor speech areas since no disruption of these outputs could be shown.

Spectrographic analysis showed that the patient's speech differed from a control group of four normal male speakers. The patient's voice was monotonous and lacked the inflection of the control group's voices. The analysis supported Jurgens and Von Cremon's subjective judgement concerning lack of expressiveness in their patient's voice.

Jurgens and Von Cremon recognized the difficulty of attributing these speech deficits to the ACG in the presence of other structural damage. Based on the following observations, however, they concluded that this patient's deficit in speech initiative and the monotone quality were primarily the result of the ACG lesion as:

1. Anterior cingulate lesions produce mutism and this blocks the volitional control of emotional utterance. Initially, all speech is prevented due to the mutism following such a lesion; therefore, emotionality through speech is also blocked.
2. The patient suffered a unilateral lesion of the left SMA but a bilateral lesion of the anterior cingulate cortex. As his vocal initiation and intonational deficits are permanent, it is more likely that these are the results of the bilateral and not the unilateral lesions.
3. Due to its rich connections with other limbic structures, the ACG is in a position especially well suited for control of emotional behaviour.
4. Monkeys conditioned to vocalize were unable to do so after ablation of the anterior cingulate cortex. The SMA was left intact in these animals, however (p. 245).

That this patient displayed neither dysarthria nor dysphonia suggested to these researchers that the ACG is not involved in motor speech planning. Instead, Jurgens and Von Cremon proposed that this brain area appears to operate as a 'drive controlling mechanism which determines, by its activity, the readiness to phonate as well as the degree of expressiveness of an emotional vocal utterance' (p. 246). These researchers do not acknowledge the possibility that readiness to phonate is an inherent part of motor speech planning and that the ACG is crucial to the successfulness of the initial step in the act of motor speech encoding.

Interestingly, although voluntary utterances were at first lost and only minimally regained by this patient, involuntary emotional vocalizations, such as moaning due to pain, were left intact. These observations serve to support Joseph's (1982) belief concerning limbic control of involuntary vocalizations in infants, children, and adults.

The cingulate gyrus then is very involved with both the initiation of vocalization as well as the emotional expression carried by vocalization. On a broader scale Smythies (1970) believes that the anterior cingulate area is the point at which emotion exerts its effect on motor acts (so blame your ACG when you miss that free throw that you made 98 out of a 100 times in your driveway but missed as the winning point in that championship game).

More recent evidence also demonstrates rich limbic input into the ACG. Amaral et al. (1993) discuss the rich connections between the amygdala and the ACG. Via the amygdala as well as the basal ganglia emotionally based learned responses have clear access to the structure responsible for the initiation of vocalization. Laryngeal tonic blocks, in which the patient is unable to phonate due to either hypo or hyper adduction of the vocal folds, may originate at this limbic cortical interface. In addition, the hippocampus has both direct and indirect input into the ACG (Nolte, 1993). This important speech area therefore has communication with both emotional and memory centres that have been shown to interfere with a variety of smooth fine motor acts, including speech. As presented earlier, the recent work of Jurgens and Zwirer (1997) points specifically to connections between the ACG and the PAG of the midbrain as points of input of emotionality into speech through the PAG's control over the vocal folds.

The anterior cingulate gyrus, then, is a critical structure in the discussion of limbic involvement and stuttering.

The thalamus

'In the thalamus, that large neuronal mass at the rostral end of the mesencephalon, it is said, lies the key to the cerebral cortex' (Walker, 1966: p. 1). The thalamus receives and sends all sensory impulses going to the cerebral cortex. It is the great switching station of the brain. The thalamus not only sends information and is responsible for the general and selective activation of far-brain sites but it has reciprocal connections with those sites. This reciprocity of communication is achieved via profuse corticothalamic fibres (Guyton, 1976; Bard, 1961). In this respect, the thalamus not only projects its influence to the cerebral cortex but is also able to monitor and appraise the results of those influences. Although the exact function of these corticothalamic fibres is not known, it is hypothesized they play a major role in the development of sensory experience and in the ability to appraise such experiences (Bard, 1961). One should note that, even though the thalamus has rich connections with the cortex, fibres from the left side of the thalamus do not cross over to the right side.

The thalamus is 'the main entryway for essentially all sensory nervous signals to the cortex' (Guyton, 1976: p. 731). Somatic signals as well as visual, auditory, and taste signals pass through the thalamus on the way to appropriate areas of the cerebral cortex. In the thalamus their specific functions of relay are served by specific thalamic nuclei and are appropriately termed *specific nuclei* of the thalamus. Their connections to specific cerebral areas are termed the 'specific thalamocortical system' (Guyton, 1976).

In addition to this specific thalamocortical system, there is a separate system, partly dependent on the first, termed the *diffuse thalamocortical system.* This coexisting system arises from diffuse thalamic nuclei and projects by diffuse fibre connections to the cortex. These nuclei are termed 'diffuse' because, unlike the nuclei of the specific system, they are not collected into specific areas; they lie between specific nuclei or on the surface of the thalamus. The fibres are termed 'diffuse' because, if they are stimulated, the result is a widespread conduction to the cerebral cortex (Gatz, 1970). It is through these systems that the thalamus can cause general or specific activation of the cerebral cortex. In addition, one class of diffuse reticular nuclei activates specific nuclei within the thalamus as well as the basal ganglia and the hypothalamus.

The thalamus is not only influential in terms of sensory impulses but is also involved in the complex processes of speech and language. Stimulation of the ventrolateral nucleus of the thalamus results in definite effects on the speech of conscious patients. The effects take two forms: either speech and voicing is arrested or the patient's speech is accelerated (Guiot, Hertzog, Rondot and Molina, 1961; Hassler, 1966). Guiot, fellow researchers, and Hassler view this response as a possible result of stimulation of the SMA via the ventrolateral nucleus. These authors qualify their results, however. Due to the proximity of the internal capsule or to conduction spread to the capsule or other adjacent structures, they could not be absolutely positive that the effects on speech were unrelated to the inexact points of stimulation. Although their results are questionable, it is known that the thalamus projects directly to the SMA via the pedunculus thalami superior tract (Penfield and Roberts, 1959; Jonas, 1982). Direct stimulation of the SMA also produces notable effects in the speech of conscious patients. This stimulation results in halted speech, significantly distorted speech, repetition of words or syllables, or hesitations and slurring of speech (Penfield and Roberts, 1959).

The thalamus has direct connections with Wernicke's area via the pulvinar and nucleus lateralis and with Broca's area via the centrum medianum (Penfield and Roberts, 1959). Thus, the thalamus acts as a functional bridge between the language area and its motor speech expression. According to Penfield and Roberts these connections 'make possible a functional interrelationship between the anterior and posterior cortical speech areas' (p. 207).

Traditionally, aphasias have primarily been attributed to damage to either Wernicke's or Broca's area. However, aphasias that, by their symptoms, parallel Broca's and Wernicke's aphasias, may be caused by damage to the thalamus alone (Penfield and Roberts, 1959; Jonas, 1982; Kirshner and Kistler, 1982). These types of speech and language difficulties typically result from insult to the left side of the thalamus or to the SMA (Penfield and Roberts, 1959; Jonas, 1982). It is much more unusual for aphasia to result from a right-sided thalamic lesion, although there are reports of this in the literature (Kirshner and Kistler, 1982). That damage to the thalamus alone can result in aphasias highlights the functional arrangements among these structures. Apparently, damage to the thalamus results in loss of the necessary integration between these cortical speech and language areas (Penfield and Roberts, 1959).

The following studies incorporate this investigative model, which, although supported, is not the only explanation of the relationship among the thalamus and speech and language. Ojemann and Ward (1971), reviewing the studies by Penfield and Roberts (1959) and Ojemann, Fedio and Van Buren (1968), hypothesized that the speech influences of the thalamus were localized in the lateral thalamic nuclei, specifically the ventrolateral nuclei. Their results were obtained from stereotaxic stimulation of the ventrolateral nuclei in 58 surgical patients. *Anomia,* defined by the authors as the inability to name an object correctly although the patient evidences no other speech difficulties, was evoked in four out of 13 patients during stimulation of the left ventrolateral nucleus in all 58 patients.

Ojemann and Ward (1971) considered anomia and perseveration to be the result of stimulating two pathways that run through the ventrolateral nucleus, the anterior centrum medianum tract and the enpassant fibres of the dorsomedial nucleus of the thalamus. They noted that their results parallel and support the hypothesis of integrative thalamic function put forth by Penfield and Roberts (1959). In addition, Ojemann, Fedio and Van Buren (1968) reported an initial inhibition of respiration followed by a prolonged expiration due to left ventrolateral thalamic stimulation. They suggest that this area may be responsible for the controlled expiration necessary for vocalization.

Additional support for the Penfield and Roberts model of thalamic integrative function may be found in the results obtained by Ciemins (1970). Ciemins reported the speech and language deficits resulting from left posterior thalamic haemorrhage in two patients. The first patient, a 53-year-old right-handed male, was admitted to the hospital because of confusion. He called familiar people and places by strange and inappropriate names. Upon neurological examination, he had difficulty naming objects and could not follow commands. There were no cranial nerve abnormalities. A formal examination for aphasia revealed a decrease in spontaneous speech, difficulty in carrying out complex commands, difficulty in writing and a deficit in the ability to read what he had been able to write. He was diagnosed as suffering from a mild mixed aphasia.

Following his death from an embolism, he was found to have had a haemorrhage involving all of the thalamic nuclei of the left side of the thalamus. This haemorrhage did not invade the internal capsule or the ventricular system. In addition, he had a microscopic lesion of the right thalamus involving the medial portion of the right ventrolateral nucleus and anterior pulvinar.

The second case of thalamic haemorrhage resulting in an aphasia is that of a 61-year-old female. Her handedness was not recorded. She was described as alert and oriented but suffering from an expressive aphasia. A formal aphasia examination was not completed. Following her death, autopsy revealed that pressure had reduced the size of the internal capsule laterally as well as the posterior aspects of the left thalamic nuclei. The lesion extended to the third ventricle through the substance of the centrum medianum. The centrum medianum is the tract identified by Penfield and Roberts (1959) as providing a link between the thalamus and Broca's area.

After reviewing these and other cases cited in the literature, Ciemins (1970) concluded that lesions involving the dominant thalamus, especially its posterior aspect, may result in aphasia. His review revealed that these thalamic aphasias are usually of a mixed type and are described as mild to moderate in severity. Ciemins offers three possible explanations for the thalamically induced aphasia:

1. As presented by Penfield and Roberts (1959), the thalamus acts as an integrator between Broca's and Wernicke's areas. Damage to the dominant side of the thalamus results in a loss of communication and integration between the cortical speech and language centres.
2. Lesions of the thalamus may result in the interruption of centrencephalic fibres necessary for activation of both the thalamus and the cortex. Interruption may result in a lack of activation of those thalamic and cortical areas necessary for speech and language.
3. It is possible that the thalamus itself has a primary speech function that, when lost, results in these aphasias.

It is also now known that areas of the thalamus, anterior cingulate gyrus and cerebellum are activated milliseconds before the onset of speech (Borden and Harris, 1982). This would certainly suggest that these areas – including the thalamus – are necessary for initiation and speech readiness.

A recent report by Abe, Yokoyama and Yorifuji (1993) describes the effects of an infarct in the paramedian region of the thalamus and midbrain. A speech disorder characterized by repetitions of the initial syllable resulted from this unfortunate event. Based on the nature of the repetitions, the authors were able to distinguish the speech problem from that of palilalia. Since the symptoms were not indicative of true stuttering or palilalia the authors termed the speech 'stuttering like repetitions' (p. 1025). Based on the anatomical evidence, Abe et al. concluded that the lesion interrupted the projections from the thalamus and midbrain to the SMA. They based this conclusion on the fact that lesions of both the SMA and basal ganglia can result in repetitive initial syllable productions similar to the repetitions produced by their patient. They consider the SMA to play a crucial role in the initiation and control of speech since lesions there produce the stuttering-like speech they describe. The lesion described in their patient interrupted the projection system from the thalamus, midbrain and the cerebellum to the SMA thus depriving that motor area of necessary input from these areas and resulting in the lack of control over speech that they felt was the ultimate cause of their patient's problem. When you pair this information with the information from Borden and Harris (1982) that reported that the thalamus and cerebellum activate milliseconds before speech onset as well as with the Jurgens and Von Cremon data showing that ACG also activates prior to speech initiation you can see that the conclusions of Abe et al. certainly make sense. If the projection pathway from the cerebellum and thalamus is interrupted then the cortical areas including the ACG and SMA are disadvantaged from the input from those cerebellar and subcortical structures. Without that information, those cortical areas are unable to exert the control that would result in smooth initiation and flow of speech.

The above data certainly suggest a definite thalamic role in the initiation and maintenance of fluent speech. This is not surprising as long as one expands the responsibility of the thalamus from a major sensory input structure to a much larger role of projection and integration of motor planning and sensory input into that activity. A report by Bhatnager and Andy (1989) supports the view that the thalamus is involved in the production of both fluent and stuttered speech. These authors discuss the case of a 61-year-old male with a long history of trigeminal pain. Previous treatments included three trigeminal rhizotomies as well as administration of the medication Sansert. A rhizotomy is a procedure that sections a nerve to relieve pain. Sansert is a drug whose action mimics that of serotonin by constricting blood vessels. It is prescribed to prevent migraine headaches. In the case of this patient it was used as an attempt to prevent blood-vessel constriction associated with the trigeminal pain. It had to be stopped, however, due to serious side effects involving his kidneys. Another rhizotomy was not attempted as he had had three such procedures previously with little positive effect. One of the cumulative effects of these treatments was a pronounced and significant stutter characterized by what these authors described as predictable sound prolongations and tonic blocks. The patient was reported to have stuttered on 58 out of 172 words. There were no secondary behaviours and no adaptation effect was demonstrated. The authors considered the stutter to be a neurological stutter for the reasons cited above and because the patient had no history of a speech problem prior to the drug and surgical interventions.

The patient's pain was treated by stereotactically implanting a chronic stimulation electrode into the left centrum medianum nucleus of his thalamus. SPECT scans revealed a significant metabolic increase in the thalamus bilaterally as a result of the electrical stimulations. There was no such increase noted at the cortical level. Within weeks of the daily electrical stimulations to control his pain the patient noticed a significant reduction in his stuttering. After eight weeks the stuttering had all but vanished.

The authors stated that these observations led them to believe that cortically produced motor speech planning is integrated via subcortical structures such as the thalamus. This integration includes that required for fluency, accuracy of synchronized motor speech commands and continuity of rhythm. They consider other associated areas of the brainstem to be involved in these activities. The present discussion would suggest that these other brainstem areas include the periaqueductal grey of the midbrain as well as the neocerebellum. The specific contributions of these areas will be detailed a little later in the text but keep Bhatnager and Andy's findings in mind when you come to those sections.

Despite reports such as that above, there is no definitive answer to the role of the thalamus in speech and language. Specific thalamic lesions that do not involve or influence other structures that may also influence speech are rare, and this lack of lesion specificity obscures conclusions as to the specific role of the thalamus in these functions. Although, without qualification, we cannot specifically state the thalamic role in speech and language, stimulation and lesion reports strongly suggest a definitive thalamic role in speech and language functioning. Further, the thalamus receives input from the amygdala and limbic system through the anterior nuclei and may act as a relay station to communicate emotional output to far cerebral sites and to Broca's and Wernicke's areas, much in the same way as it acts as a functional bridge between these areas. One could also argue that it is at the thalamus, in addition to other areas, where limbic input is added to the communication between these classic speech/language areas. We need to keep abreast of research into this really fascinating structure in order to apply those data to our knowledge of both fluency and stuttering.

The right cerebral hemisphere and its influence on speech and language

One of many responsibilities of the left hemisphere, in most individuals, is the speech and language function of Broca's and Wernicke's areas. Traditionally, the right hemisphere has been assigned the musical facilities such as rhythm and melody, the analysis of spatial relationships, the ability to holistically perceive objects and facts and the ability to graphically copy figures (Ross and Mesulam, 1979). However, the right hemisphere may also be the dominant hemisphere for certain linguistic contributions to speech.

Neurological examinations of left-hemisphere lesions have shown that aphasias result from damage to Broca's area, Wernicke's area or to both areas, thus assigning the left hemisphere responsibility for the production of speech and the comprehension of language. By contrast, the right hemisphere has been credited with little or no influence over the production of speech or the comprehension of language. The dominance of the left hemisphere in speech and language has been based on the evaluation of the vocabulary, syntax, and articulation of language. This view has not fully taken into account other aspects of speech, such as prosody and gesturing, which overlie and accompany speech. These two influences 'are crucial for allowing spoken language to acquire emotional and thus affective tone' (Ross and Mesulam, 1979: p. 144).

Ross defines 'prosody' as the melodious aspect of speech that is the result of variations in pitch, rhythm, and stresses in articulation that produce additional semantic meaning and emotional meaning in speech. 'Gestures' on the other hand, are movements that 'accompany, emphasize and colour speech' (p. 147). This definition of gesturing excludes pantomiming, in which the entire idea or proposition is conveyed to the receiver. In this context, a gesture is that flip of the hand that augments the individual's verbalization of indifference. Gesturing is a spontaneous accompaniment to speech. Pantomime is propositional in that it may be used in place of speech to express an entire idea or thought.

In a series of three articles, Ross and Mesulam (1979), Ross (1981) and Ross, Harney, DeLacoste Utamsing and Purdy (1981) review and discuss the results of damage to two areas of the right hemisphere. They evaluated their patients using traditional neurological examination, clinical observation, computer tomography scans, and autopsy results. The two areas of damage to the right hemispheres of these patients mirrored the location of Broca's and Wernicke's areas on the left cortex.

The researchers classify damage to the areas of the right cortex using the general term aprosodias. *Aprosodia* refers to the loss of the affective emotional component of speech and gesturing (Ross et al., 1981). Additional support for these findings may be found in the work of Larsen and Lassen (1978). These researchers reported that measures of regional blood flow during automatic speech tasks resulted in blood flow on the right hemisphere that was homologous to that observed in the left hemisphere. In both hemispheres blood flow was increased to the SMA, the inferior sensorimotor strip and an area of the posterior-superior temporal lobe. In the next chapter we shall see that results of PET scans and more recent cerebral blood flow data also support Ross and his findings with definite implications for stuttering.

Ross and associates (1981) reported that damage to the right hemisphere's anterior centre results in deficits of spontaneous gesturing as well as deficits of emotional input into speech. The result is very flat, monotonous, unemotional input into speech production. Ross termed this type of aprosodia 'motor aprosodia'. Conversely, a lesion to the posterior area of the right temporal lobe resulted in a deficit in the ability to decode emotional affect in the speech or gestures of others. This deficit, analogous to damage to Wernicke's area, has been termed 'sensory aprosodia' (Ross et al., 1981).

Accepting the left hemisphere as being responsible for the propositional components of speech and language and the right hemisphere as being responsible for the affective emotional components of speech and gesturing raises the question of how the brain integrates these co-existing systems. Ross and associates (1981) have addressed this question in relation to their findings and inferences concerning the aprosodias. They cite a case of motor aprosodia occurring in a 47-year-old male, who later succumbed to his injuries. An autopsy revealed that the right-sided infarction involved the posterior two-thirds of the anterior limb, the entire genu, and the anterior third of the posterior limb of the rostral internal capsule. It is important to note the lesion was confined to the white matter and was located within the internal capsule 'below the corticocortical transcallosal connections' (p. 747). The right hemisphere lesion destroyed almost all motor output from this hemisphere and 'correlated well with the left hemiplegia presented by this patient' (p. 747). Autopsy also revealed 'a left sided lesion that was small and clinically silent' (p. 747) as there were no pseudobulbar symptoms or other findings consistent with a previous stroke.

The results of this single case led Ross and associates to postulate that actual 'motor integration of the language outputs from each hemisphere takes place in a subcortical site below the level of the deep telencephalic nuclei' (p. 747). If this motor integration were transcallosal, the patient should not have presented a motor aprosodia since the lesion did not involve transcallosal connections. That is not to say that no integration is transcallosal. There is occasional transient mismatching between propositional speech and emotional overlay in patients following transection of the cerebral commissures. This usually resolves itself after two post-operative weeks.

Although the authors were unable to be more specific regarding the exact location or tract responsible for the emotional and motor speech point of interface, there are several points of transcortical communication. As mentioned previously, there are the major transcallosal commissures. There are, according to Ross at al. (1981), subcortical connections between the bilateral amygdalas and hippocampi. Lastly, the work of Jones and Powell (1970) suggests that, in humans, input from the limbic system, which has bilateral connections, travels into Broca's area via the mediodorsal thalamic nuclei. One might infer that communication from the right hemisphere that is integrated with speech as the emotionally loaded suprasegmentals may be the result of limbic transcortical connections.

It would appear, then, that speech, language and their emotional and gestural overlay are the results of interaction and integration between the two hemispheres. Input to Ross's anterior area of the right hemisphere from the limbic system is translated into the emotionality conveyed by inflections and prosodies of speech. In addition, there may also be input, via the thalamus, from the limbic system directly into Broca's area of the left hemisphere. Comprehension of emotionality and gesturing may be the result of interactions of Ross's posterior area of the right hemisphere and limbic structures. In any event, in a very real sense, and both expressively and receptively, speech and language can be regarded as brain-wide functions and not the sole responsibility of the left hemisphere.

Looking at the above information raises an interesting hypothesis: could the fluency-enhancing action of delayed auditory feedback be explained through this information? In delayed auditory feedback the speaker's words are slightly delayed in being heard by that speaker. For many fluent speakers this results in dysfluency of their ongoing speech while for those who stutter this often results in a slowed droned but fluent monotone. Now, in the past this fluency was explained through audition, but the above information may provide an additional explanation. Could it be that the delay results in fluency because the prosodic contribution from the anterior area of Ross on the right is somehow blocked by the delayed auditory feedback? Or could it be that the area is simply never activated due to the delayed feedback? After all, the effect of the delay for someone who stutters is fluent but monotonous speech. Monotone has to be either the result of an activation or – more to this point – the result of a non-activation. It could well be that the auditory effect coupled with the attention that must be paid to slowing down one's speech to match the effect of the delay may serve to allow only left hemisphere speech control which, similar to the effect of damage to the anterior area of Ross, results in little or no prosodic overlay from the right hemisphere. No (or very little) right-hemisphere input into speech may then result in a fluent monotone.

Remember, too, that one problem encountered by some therapies for stuttering involve what is termed 'speech naturalness'. This is simply more prosody than fluent monotone in the speech of those treated for stuttering. However, this is precisely what is so troublesome for many treated individuals. When attempting to sound more 'natural', i.e. more prosodic, the fluency breaks down and stuttering emerges. It could be that this is occurring because the right-hemisphere prosodic centres and the subcortical emotional areas that serve them re-establish their inappropriate amounts of input into the production of speech by the dominant left hemisphere. This will be explored further in the chapter reviewing neuroimaging and stuttering.

The concept of an emotional motor system

It has long been known that the left side of the face conveys more motor-based emotional expression than does the right. This is due to the innervation of that side of the face by the contralateral right hemisphere. Also, from the above discussion of the aprosodias, the right hemisphere has other efferent and afferent contributions to speech. Through the amygdala and hippocampus – the so-called temporal limbic system – there is influence over laryngeal and respiratory sub-systems of speech. These and many other findings led Ross (1996) to explore the validity of the presence of an emotional motor system, the EMS. He concluded that there is, in fact, evidence to support such a system. In his schema, the EMS emanates from the limbic structures and runs in parallel with the cortical motor systems. More study is necessary before the presence of such a system can be shown empirically but the idea in a context such as this is tantalizing to say the least. An EMS would explain emotional disruption of learned behaviours so much more elegantly and simply than connectionist explanations, such as the present one attempts to do.

The supplementary motor area

The supplementary motor area (SMA) is located on the superior medial aspect of both frontal lobes anterior to the premotor cortices (Penfield and Roberts, 1959; Wiesendanger, 1981; Nolte, 1993). The SMA has many connections with cortical and subcortical areas. The SMA has efferent and afferent connections with the thalamus via the pedunculus thalami superior tract (Penfield and Roberts, 1959). The anterior cingulate gyrus receives input from the entire limbic system and in turn projects profusely to the SMA. In addition, via the basal ganglia, the amygdala has input into the SMA (Damasio, 1984). It has been hypothesized that the SMA of the dominant hemisphere connects with Broca's area by looping through the hypothalamus. It may also be that this connection provides additional limbic input to Broca's area through the connecting loop (Botez and Barbeau, 1971).

Through cortical stimulation studies, Penfield and Roberts (1959) demonstrated that the SMA of the dominant hemisphere contributed to the motor speech output of Broca's area. Electrical stimulation of the SMA resulted in distortions, hesitations, and repetitions in the ongoing speech of their conscious patients. The results were so striking that Penfield and Roberts designated the SMA as the 'third speech centre' (p. 202) and referred to Broca's area and Wernicke's area as the major cortical speech and language areas.

The connections between the SMA and Broca's area, with the cingulate gyrus, the amygdala via the basal ganglia, and the hypothalamus, suggest that the SMA contributes to the suprasegmental variables that transmit the emotional quality of speech. The SMA also appears to contribute to movements that reflect emotionality. Recent evidence supports this inference. Damasio (1984) reports that a lesion of the SMA of the dominant hemisphere results in the 'SMA syndrome'. Behavioural manifestations of the SMA syndrome include diminished speech, diminished gestural accompaniment with speech, and emotional facial paralysis. Emotional facial paralysis refers to lack of facial movement reflective of the individual's emotions. If the patient laughs, smiles or cries there is facial movement only on the side of the face contralateral to the SMA lesion. If the lesion is bilateral, the manifestations are, of course, permanent.

The SMA of the left hemisphere connects with Broca's area of the same side. The SMA of the right hemisphere connects with the homologous area of Broca's on the right. This is the anterior area of Ross (Ross et al., 1981), which appears to supply the prosodic overlay to motor speech. The bilateral SMAs communicate with one another via the corpus callosum. It is this commissure that allows the right-hemisphere SMA to assume the responsibilities of a lesioned left hemisphere SMA. Prosodic disturbances are not described in the literature as a function of SMA electrical stimulation. Therefore, the SMA of the dominant side may act as one relay between the anterior areas of Ross and Broca. As suggested previously, these connections may be from the anterior area of Ross to the right side of the thalamus, subcortically. The right side of the thalamus connects with the left hemisphere SMA, Broca's area, and Wernicke's area (Damasio, 1984a; Penfield and Roberts, 1959).

Electrical stimulation of the SMA in conscious patients is reported to most often result in vocalization, or in hesitations, repetitions and distortions of ongoing speech (Penfield and Roberts, 1959). More recent stimulation studies, however, have shown a quite different action of the SMA on speech. Damasio (1984a) reports that if the SMA of the dominant side is stimulated at the moment of speech onset, a complete arrest of vocalization and motor speech results. Patients report complete helplessness at any attempt to circumvent the arrest.

More recent evidence concerning the SMA consolidates the contributions of this area to speech production. Connor and Abbs (1990) describe the inputs from the basal ganglia into the SMA via the thalamus. In this model the SMA as previously discussed acts as a functional bridge between the basal ganglia and the primary motor cortex. Further, regional blood flow studies shows activation of the SMA before the onset of movements. The SMA is only activated during tasks requiring fine motor movement, sequential control such as is seen in movements of the foot, hand, or the articulators (Connor and Abbs, 1990). It will come as no surprise, then, to learn that regional blood flow studies of Warburton et al. (1996) demonstrated activation of the SMA and anterior cingulate gyrus during noun and verb retrieval tasks.

One of the more interesting ideas put forth about the SMA, in addition to other cortical areas, is that the area is an evolutionary extension of the limbic lobe (Goldberg, 1985). In this model the argument is made that there are two motor programming systems: the medial composed of the cingulate and the SMA both with an evolutionary origin in the hippocampus and a lateral, composed of the arcuate premotor area with an evolutionary origin in the piraform cortex. In this schema, the SMA has significant projections to the primary motor cortex responsible for the leg, arm, and face; cortical relationships with Brodman's area 6, the medial-dorsolateral prefrontal area and the cingulate gyrus. The basal ganglia are the area of SMA subcortical dependence. The arcuate system has significant projections to the primary motor cortex responsible for the arm and face; cortical relationships with a variety of areas including frontoparietal operculum, insula, auditory association cortex, and the visual and somatic fields. The area of this system's subcortical dependence is the cerebellum.

One important contribution of the SMA in this model is the intermediary role it would play between the drive-controlling aspects of the anterior cingulate gyrus (remember that the man with damage to his anterior cingulate gyrus lost the drive but not the ability to repeat speech) and the selection and execution of specific movements or strategies of movement. The SMA would be expected to perform this service due to its location between the anterior cingulate gyrus and the primary motor cortex. Goldberg considers the SMA to be a 'proto-motor paralimbic cortex located at the confluence of anterior cingulate, superior mesial prefrontal, dorsolateral area 6, and mesial primary motor cortex' (p. 576). According to Goldberg, the SMA is part of the cortico-limbic-reticular system and serves to focus limbic input into motor areas. One would assume then that it would serve to direct limbic input into those cortical areas responsible for speech, given the speech responsibilities of the SMA Thus, this area presents yet another location for major limbic input into the speech process.

Neurophysiological data concerning the SMA suggest that the SMA is an important area with respect to emotional expression. Damage results not only in less speech and gesture but also in monotone speech. Accompanying this deficit is lack of facial, labial and emotional expression contralateral to the lesion (Damasio, 1984). Finally, stimulation of the SMA may result not only in vocalization or adverse effects on motor speech (Penfield and Roberts, 1959) but may also result in arrest of vocalization and speech (Damasio, 1984). It may be inferred, then, that the SMA of the dominant side joins the areas and structures previously discussed as critical to normal speech production, capable of disruption of fluent motor speech, and contributing to facial emotional expression accompanying speech.

The most recent information published on the SMA was in the February 1998 edition of *Nature*. Fried, Wilson, MacDonald and Behnke reported the results of electrical stimulation of the lateral border of the SMA. The patient was undergoing an evaluation of her epilepsy when she suddenly began light laughter in the absence of humorous stimuli. When asked during each episode of stimulated laughter what was making her laugh, the patient ascribed humour to various different aspects of the situation, none of which was obvious in amusement value. For instance, she said 'you guys are just so funny . . . standing around'. The duration and intensity of the laughter increased with increasing levels of electrical stimulation. The authors concluded that the anterior portion of the SMA is 'part of a further development in humans to accommodate the specialized functions of speech, manual dexterity and laughter' (p. 650).

The Cerebellum

The cerebellum has traditionally been thought to be primarily, if not exclusively, responsible for co-ordination and control of movement. There is a growing body of evidence, however, that is greatly expanding the role of this apparently underestimated structure. In the face of the dramatic effects that damage to the cerebellum has on movement control this lack of appreciation of other contributions may be understood. Recent findings, however, demonstrate that this structure contributes not just to movement efficiency and accuracy but also to the learning of movements and acquisition of conditioned responses – especially conditioned fear responses. It also has both direct and indirect reciprocal connections with the limbic system through the hypothalamus, but also communicates to the anterior frontal lobe and Broca's area as well as receiving input from the temporal lobe auditory areas – especially from Wernicke's area. The cerebellar connections via the thalamus to left-hemisphere speech and language areas are through the left ventrolateral nucleus.

In the past the cerebellum was not considered to be involved in motor learning but was regarded as being of primary importance for motor performance. Before the use of specific neurotoxin delivery methods it had been impossible to test the contribution of the cerebellum to learning. The destruction of areas of the cerebellum resulted in such motoric deficits that any learning problems that might have developed were impossible to investigate. The ability to deliver neurotoxins specific for certain nerve cells to very specific areas of the cerebellum resulted in a classic study by Watson and McElligott (1984). These researchers taught various mazes to a set of rats. When certain nuclei of the rats' cerebellums were destroyed by the toxin it was found that they were as mobile and as co-ordinated as the untreated rats but it was also seen that they were no longer able to negotiate the maze that they had shown such proficiency at solving before the procedure. While their motor abilities were spared, their performance of a learned motor behaviour was severely impaired. All other areas of their brains were intact.

The cerebellum is also very involved in the learning of conditioned responses, especially instrumental responses that are fear based. (Remember this when you get to the next chapter on the limbic system and learning.) Selective lesioning of the cerebellar cortex, area HVI, that projects to the interpositus nuclei, will impair or even extinguish a conditioned instrumental response (Lalonde and Botez,1990).

Electrical stimulation of the cerebellum will also result in overt manifestations of emotionality. Animals with lesioned cerebellums will show rage behaviour, attack behaviour, and behaviours associated with fear reactions. None of that is surprising as the cerebellum has reciprocal connections with the hypothalamus and through it to the rest of the limbic system (Lalonde and Botez, 1990).

In 1991, Leiner, Leiner and Dow published a review of evolutionary development of the cerebellum, reciprocal connections of the cerebellum with the thalamus, limbic system and cortex, and the contributions of the cerebellum to computation, cognition, and speech and language.

As the human brain enlarged so, too, did the cerebellum. This development of the cerebellum proceeded in parallel with the development of the expanding cerebral association areas, particularly those of the enlarging frontal lobes. This cerebellar development went so well, in fact, that at the present time our cerebellums contain more neurones than our cerebral cortexes. A great deal of attention has, of course, been paid to the development of the cerebrum, but the development of the cerebellum also needs appreciation. Just as new areas evolved in the cerebrum, new areas also evolved in the cerebellum. One can correctly refer to these newly developed areas of the cerebellum as the 'neocerebellum', just as those newly developed areas of the cerebrum are referred to as the 'neocortex'.

This new development can be seen especially in the lateral aspects of the cerebellum. This area of the cerebellum developed new connections to the evolving neocortex in order to serve evolving skills made possible by that evolution. One such emerging skill was the development of human speech and language functions. Therefore, new connections via enlarged areas of the brainstem allowed connections between the anterior frontal lobes, the posterior temporal lobes and the lateral portions of the neocerebellum. In our present brains, the neocerebellum serves several speech and language functions. First, it acts as a link between Broca's area in the frontal lobe and Wernicke's area in the temporal. Leiner, Leiner, and Dow say that the neocerebellum serves as an additional association area, not only able to contribute to motor speech but also able to contribute to cognitive processes that think of the words to be said. This position is supported by neuroimaging studies cited by the authors that demonstrate dramatic activation of the lateral cerebellum during word-processing tasks.

The neocerebellum's contributions to cognitive tasks can be shown by studies of unfortunate patients suffering from a variety of syndromes, tumours, stroke, or lesions of the lateral areas of the cerebellum. Individuals with Williams syndrome have a mental retardation but display verbal and linguistic skills far above their cognitive abilities. These speech and language skills include normal syntax and semantics. Magnetic resonance imaging of these children always shows characteristic signatures; their forebrains are significantly smaller than normal, their paleocerebellum is low normal but their neocerebellum, the lateral areas of the cerebellum, are normal. By contrast, children with Down syndrome show the opposite. Their forebrain is far more normal in volume but their neocerebellum is significantly reduced in size in comparison to normal children. Complex language abilities are not the norm for these children – a stark contrast to children with Williams syndrome.

At the furthest end of the continuum are those children with autism. Autistic children demonstrate a reduction in the size of the neocerebellum as well as the brainstem. There appears to be a drastic reduction in the number of nerve cells in the lateral cerebellums of these children. Although no causal relationship can be deduced, the fact that autistic children do have a characteristic deficit of the neocerebellum does point out the possible contribution of the cerebellum to social, linguistic and cognitive skills.

As with animal studies, reports of damage to the human cerebellum, especially of damage to the midline cerebellum, include rage reactions, loss of self-control, and extremely uninhibited behaviour. Total removal of this structure is always associated with cognitive, emotional and social deficits, often of catastrophic proportions.

The influences detailed above are made possible by the connections of the neocerebellum with the frontal motor areas, especially the premotor areas and Broca's area as well as connections with the limbic system. The connections to the frontal lobes are through the ventrolateral and central lateral nuclei of the thalamus. According to Leiner, Leiner and Dow, the route via the ventrolateral nucleus is the more direct of the two. Fibres target specific areas in the prefrontal cortex. The lateral prefrontal cortex is an association area comprised of Brodman's areas eight through 12 and, notable for this discussion, areas 44 through 47. Areas 44 and 45 both include part of Broca's area. The authors consider these two areas to have both motor and cognitive contributions to language. This language function is demonstrated during stereotaxic electrical stimulation of the ventrolateral nucleus. This results in linguistic deficits, such as naming errors, as long as the electrical current is maintained. These deficits were not motoric – they were not due to articulatory errors; these were ideational errors – language based mistakes. Leiner, Leiner, and Dow state that because the ventrolateral projections originating in the neocerebellum 'can reach cortical areas that are involved in some cognitive functions as well as motor functions (e.g. Broca's area), these projections provide an anatomical substrate through which the lateral cerebellum can contribute to cognitive functions, including language' (p. 122). The central lateral nucleus provides a less direct route and is more diffuse in target areas. It is considered to allow involvement of the cerebellum in cortical alertness, attention, and arousal.

Via the hypothalamus, the neocerebellum has direct reciprocal connections with the limbic system. A less direct route to limbic structures is provided through the brainstem reticular areas and structures. Connections such as these are the reason for the rage reactions seen in patients with lesions of cerebellar areas. The reciprocity of these limbic connections and the input from the cerebellum into both right and left hemisphere frontal lobe motor areas is very interesting in light of neuroimaging studies to be reviewed in the next chapter. One of the best of these studies reported cerebellar activations twice those of normal controls in the stuttering subjects during a stuttering event. Given the connections that the neocerebellum has with limbic structures and frontal motor areas, including Broca's area (and, presumably, the anterior of Ross on the right hemisphere) such an activation increase is understandable.

Summary

Results of electrical stimulation and lesion studies suggest cortical and subcortical areas that appear to be involved in emotionally originated motoric disruptions of speech. It is not suggested that all of the motoric, respiratory, or laryngeal responses capable of being elicited by these structures occur in each individual who stutters. Behaviours manifested as stuttering may be very individualized. From this standpoint, the results of electrical stimulation and lesion studies provide a repertoire of disruptions from which individual manifestations of the disorder may develop. In order to facilitate appreciation of the extent of these disruptions in those readers less familiar with the neurological information presented, a synopsis of the preceding results of lesion and stimulation follows.

Amygdala

1. Connects with the contralateral amygdala, thalamus, cingulate gyrus and other limbic areas as well as the cortex and basal ganglia.
2. Activation results in interactions with the hippocampus, which allows conditioned reflex formation to occur.
3. Activation can result in either clonic or tonic movements of the eyes, head, face or jaw.
4. Activation can also result in rhythmic movements of the jaw and tongue.
5. Stimulation in human beings also results in reports of unaccountable fear, supporting the contention of the limbic basis of internal emotional states.
6. Serves to activate or inhibit actions of the hypothalamus, which is responsible for physiological manifestations of emotions.
(For a complete list of amygdala connections within the central nervous system see the appendix.)

Hypothalamus

1. Activation can result in stimulation of the premotor cortex, which is responsible for facial expression, facial movements, chewing, and swallowing.
2. Activation can result in tonic arrest of movements originated by the primary motor area.

3. Indirectly activates the supplementary motor areas via the premotor cortex, which results in distortions, hesitations, or repetitions of speech.
4. Is responsible for cardiovascular changes that accompany internal states of emotion (the flight or fight physiological responses to threat or fear).
5. Lesions can result in rage behaviour supporting the limbic system as the basis of emotion.

Anterior cingulate gyrus

1. Connects with the thalamus and limbic system.
2. Has profuse connections with the supplementary motor areas. Activation of these areas results in hesitations, distortions, or repetitions in speech.
3. Activation can result in an arrest of respiration, tonic blocks of movements and/or clonic motor movements.
4. The cingulate gyrus connects with all other central nervous system areas that produce vocalization upon stimulation.
5. This area has a direct connection with the motor neurones of the larynx.
6. Lesions result in voluntary mutism.
7. This is considered to be the point at which emotion exerts its effect on motor acts.

Hippocampus

1. This has extensive connections with all parts of the limbic system, including the cingulate gyrus.
2. It receives extensive connections from the temporal neocortex.
3. It is thought to receive information about the state of the external environment and to feed this information to the limbic system as an internal representation of the external world.
4. Acting with the amygdala and other limbic structures, it is thought to be crucial for conditioned reflex formation.
5. It activates the hypothalamus for correlated visceral, cardiovascular, and other physiological changes associated with emotion.
6. It is considered crucial for laying down recent experience into long-term memory stores.
7. It appears to act as a limbic switching station, directing information to various limbic structures and, via these structures, to other subcortical and cortical areas.

Septum and septal area

1. This area receives and sends information to all parts of the limbic system, especially the hypothalamus.

2. Lesions result in aggressive rage behaviour, supporting the limbic basis of emotion.
3. Stimulation results in changes in blood pressure, pulse and respiration rates.
4. It appears to inhibit or facilitate actions of the hippocampus.

Thalamus

1. The thalamus can send and receive all sensory information to the cortex.
2. It has many connections with the limbic system and the anterior cingulate gyrus.
3. It projects to and receives fibres from the supplementary motor areas, stimulation of which results in hesitations, distortions, and repetitions in speech.
4. It acts as a functional bridge between Broca's area and Wernicke's area.
5. Stimulation can result in speech arrest or speech-rate acceleration.
6. Stimulation can result in clonic repetitions of the initial sound of the first word spoken during stimulation.
7. Lesions can result in traditional categories of aphasia.
8. The thalamus is thought to exert strong influence over the controlled expirations required for speech.

Right cerebral hemisphere

1. This has profuse connections with the limbic system.
2. It has an anterior area that mirrors the locations of Broca's area on the left and is thought to be responsible for the suprasegmental aspects of speech that carry emotional meaning.
3. It has a posterior area that mirrors the location of Wernicke's area on the left and is thought to be responsible for the interpretation of emotionality in the suprasegmentals and gestures of others.
4. At the moment of stuttering there is greater blood flow to the anterior area of the right hemisphere than to Broca's area of the left hemisphere.

Supplemental motor area (SMA)

1. Stimulation of the left SMA results in hesitations, distortions and repetitions in speech.
2. If this stimulation coincides with the initiation of speech, phonation and articulation are arrested.
3. A lesion of the SMA results in diminished speech and gestures, and in monotone speech.

4. Lesions also result in emotional facial paralysis in which the patient can smile or show types of emotional facial expressions on command but is unable to show such expressions when spontaneously accompanying emotional states.
5. It has connections with the limbic system via the anterior cingulate gyrus.
6. The SMA of the right hemisphere connects with the anterior area of that hemisphere thought to be responsible for emotion carrying suprasegmental aspects of speech and gesture.
7. SMA has connections with the amygdala via the prefrontal motor areas.
8. SMA has direct connections with the thalamus.
9. The SMA has been termed 'the third speech centre' by Penfield and Roberts (1959).

Cerebellum

1. The cerebellum has connections with Broca's area and Wernicke's area via the thalamus.
2. It acts as a functional bridge between the classic speech and language areas of the cortex.
3. It has language functions through contributions to such tasks as word finding.
4. It has reciprocal connections with the limbic system through the hypothalamus.

Finally, a word of caution is necessary. None of the authors reporting the previous neurological results were addressing the contributions to stuttering behaviour from the structures or areas under their study. Nevertheless, the results of these stimulations, ablation, or lesion studies do demonstrate responses that resemble behaviours traditionally identified with stuttering. It is proposed that the integrated actions of these cortical and subcortical structures and areas provide the underlying neurological basis of the emotional and behavioural manifestations known as stuttering.

Chapter Two
Conditioning and stuttering

As suggested in the previous chapter, stuttering – like all behaviour – has a neurophysiological basis. However, stuttering does not exist in a learning or emotional void. Individuals who stutter must learn to stutter and they must also learn the instrumental avoidance behaviours so closely associated with the tonic/clonic block complex of dysfluent behaviours. Just as the current level of neurophysiological knowledge cannot fully explain the etiology of the disorder, neither can learning theory. Learning coupled with neurophysiology can, however, present a much more complete picture of how the primary and associated behaviours are acquired and maintained.

As there are only two primary types of blocks – clonic and tonic – with, perhaps, individual variations in terms of predominance it seems reasonable to conclude that the interference with fluency from subcortical limbic areas has common manifestations. That is, there is a limited repertoire of this type of interference: either the result is a clonic block or a tonic block. One can then assume that the actual block is not learned. The type of block produced is prescribed by the underlying neurophysiology of the behaviour. How the individual deals with the expectation of the block, the moment of the block, the actuality of the block and the moments after the occurrence are learned – the block itself is neurophysiologically determined.

Accepting the above, the work of Brutten and Shoemaker (1967) and their 'two-factor theory of stuttering' is, I think, a 'best fit' here. According to this theory, it is not the actual stuttering that is learned; it is the negative emotional reaction to the act of speaking that is learned. Stuttering is often but certainly not always the result of this internal negative emotional reaction. After all, no one who stutters, no matter how severely, stutters all the time. These authors contend that the negative emotional response is learned through classical conditioning paradigms. This seemed very reasonable to Brutten and Shoemaker as they considered almost all emotional learning to be based on classical conditioning. Classical conditioning paradigms readily and elegantly explain how emotional reactions can be acquired and generalized to stimuli further removed from the original sources.

The second half of the two-factor theory explains the learning of secondary behaviours associated with stuttering. Instrumental learning is credited with the acquisition of these components of the stuttering complex. Individuals learn that dropping eye contact can result in a block being avoided, or can make it less severe, or can enable them to escape from it, so eye contact is habitually dropped when the occurrence of a stuttering event is anticipated or occurs. Over time the effectiveness of this technique reduces but does not disappear. A new, more effective behaviour is then incorporated – perhaps turning the head away from the listener. In this way a constellation of secondary behaviours surrounds the person who stutters. Interestingly, one can determine the order of acquisition of these behaviours simply by observation, as the oldest is typically performed first followed by the next and so forth. The last secondary behaviour seen is the most recent one learned. If you just suggested to yourself that these behaviours are similar to a chain with the first triggering the second, the second triggering the third and so on, you have accurately described this phenomenon.

These secondary behaviours are best explained as instrumentally learned because the person performing them believes them to be instrumental in avoiding, lessening, or escaping the block. For those readers who do not stutter or who have limited experience with secondary behaviours and instrumental learning a good example might be the scenario involving you forgetting an important birthday or your wedding anniversary – the negative emotional arousal caused by such a lapse should have resulted in your performing instrumental behaviours to avoid such an occurrence in the future, such as marking a calendar a year in advance . . . the learning of secondary behaviours for stuttering follows the same pattern, just more often. . .

The two-factor theory is also an ideal perspective from which to discuss the acquisition of learned behaviours in stuttering because it allows us to discuss classically and instrumentally learned behaviours through the activities of such structures as the amygdala, hippocampus and basal ganglia. In fact, one might be tempted to champion the two-factor theory as the concept best able to explain the learned operational aspects of stuttering behaviours.

The amygdala and conditioned fear

As you remember from Chapter One (we have to keep exercising that old hippocampus) a common reaction to electrical stimulation of the amygdala in human subjects is a feeling of deep, unaccountable fear. Animal subjects whose amygdalas have been removed show various inappropriate behaviours ranging from passiveness to oral and manual manipulation of objects that would have previously stimulated fear-based avoidance behaviours. A good example of this is an amygdalized monkey approaching a rubber snake, picking it up, putting it in its mouth and examining it manually. No self-respecting normal primate would do this either in the wild or in captivity (neither would you or I, for that matter).

Now, there is one topic that needs to be addressed before discussing specific findings regarding the role of the amygdala in fear conditioning – that of the animal subjects that are by far the most commonly used (it is after all to be expected that it might be more difficult to obtain human subjects for amygdala lesion studies. Even undergraduates enrolled in 'introduction to general psychology' might be expected to draw the line there). There are, of course, enormous differences between rats and humans. However, as Davis (1992) reminds us, there are also some very close similarities when discussing primitive responses such as fear. Davis compared the behavioural measures used to identify a fearful response in animal subjects with the DSM-III criteria for generalized anxiety and reported the following rather startling similarities:

Animals: increased heart rate
Humans: heart pounding

Animals: defecation
Humans: diarrhoea

Animals: decreased salivation
Humans: dry mouth

Animals: grooming
Humans: fidgeting

Animals: stomach ulcers
Humans: upset stomach

Animals: freezing
Humans: apprehensive expectation – a feeling that something bad is going
        to happen

Animals: respiratory change
Humans: increased respiration

Animals: urination
Humans: increased urination.

Animals: scanning and vigilance
Humans: scanning and vigilance

Animals: increased tendency to become startled
Humans: jumpiness, easy to startle

These are not perfect fits but the behaviours are close enough to enable us to draw tentative conclusions when making the leap from animal to human models.

It is also important to recall that the amygdala connects with and receives input from a wide variety of near and far brain areas and structures. For specifics please refer to the information in Chapter One and the Appendix where the currently known connections are listed. Recall that this almond-shaped structure sends input to the striatum, basal forebrain, thalamus, hypothalamus, brainstem, hippocampus, insula, cingulate gyrus, frontal, temporal, and occipital lobes. The amygdala also receives input from just as wide a variety of structures and areas. Due to these reciprocal connections and to its location, the amygdala is in a unique position to act as the area of convergence for stimuli and for classically conditioned emotional and behavioural responses. This is particularly true for classically conditioned emotional and behavioural fear responses. A large number of animal studies and a few human studies have shown that ablation of specific nuclei of the amygdala results in either an inability to learn conditioned responses or the inability to manifest those learned responses. Davis (1992) reviews a number of such studies. His conclusion, based on his own work and the previous work of others, is that the amygdala is an area of convergence of the neural activity generated by conditioned and unconditioned stimuli. Such a hypothesis is also proposed by Gloor (1997) in his updated and truly magnificent work *The Temporal Lobe and Limbic System*. In these works the authors propose that the amygdala receives both the conditioned and unconditioned stimuli. Sympathetic activation occurs through connections with the hypothalamus: cardiovascular changes, Galvanic skin responses, paleness, pupil dilation and blood pressure changes are generated. Connections with the dorsal motor nerve of the vagus and the nucleus ambiguous result in parasympathetic activations: a need to urinate, bradycardia and stomach reactions. Through the parabrachial nucleus, the amygdala can cause increased respiration or even respiratory distress. It can cause freezing behaviours through innervation to aqueductal grey of the midbrain tonic (remember that it is the aqueductal grey that figures so prominently in Denny and Smith's (1997) stuttering theory). Of particular interest here is the fact that connections with the trigeminal nerve can result in jaw and mouth movements that reflect the internal emotion of fear. Last, but certainly not least for those of us who have experienced it, the release of adrenocorticotrophic hormone (ACTH) resulting from stimulation by the amygdala and the paraventricular nucleus of the hypothalamus leads to corticosteroid release, the so-called stress response encountered so often by novice public speakers (and novice lion tamers).

In a study to be reviewed in the next chapter it is suggested that stuttering is related to dopamine levels. With this in mind it is interesting to note that Davis reports that, due to projections from the amygdala, the ventral tegmental area can mediate dopamine increases due to stress in the prefrontal cortex, an area that contributes much to voluntary motor planning and initiation. According to Davis, fear-potentiated reactions in humans show strong lateralization to the right hemisphere, perhaps due to greater participation by the right-sided amygdala.

One important aspect of human conditioning is missing in the above lists: that of cognitive contributions. According to Halgren (1992) the amygdala is in just the correct location and has the correct neocortical connections to act as the link between the cortex and the brainstem that is critical for internal emotional experience and for conditioned emotional responses. Halgren reports that a variety of studies show conclusively that the amygdala receives both high level cognitive as well as visceral inputs and that it has influence over the contents and the quality of our aware-ness as well as over the expression of autonomic states in response to external and internally generated stimuli. It is really interesting to note that, from his work and the work he reviews, the amygdala is involved in the evaluation of complex stimuli before these are evaluated cognitively. In fact, Halgren believes this occurs before these stimuli even enter our awareness. Such responsibilities certainly take the amygdala a long way past the original thought that it was primarily responsible for our sense of smell (for a truly engaging discussion of limbic responses to smell, including our own body odour and that of others, see Gloor, 1997). Such studies also support the theory of emotionality proposed by Cannon and not that of James (see Chapter One for a review of these).

Learning and conditioning depend on remembering. What we remember and what emotions we remember themselves depend upon our friend the hippocampus. It is this worm-shaped (or seahorse-shaped, depending on whom one reads) structure that is responsible for holding significant stimuli in short-term memory prior to the transfer to long-term storage. Damage to the hippocampus results in anterograde amnesia, a condition resulting in the inability to learn any non-procedurally based new information. One remembers the past prior to the lesion but one cannot remember the immediate past. The amygdala has reciprocal connections with this structure and this accounts for the memory retaining the emotion generated at the time of occurrence.

What we believe is highly influenced by what we remember. If we believe that, for us, speech is difficult, we believe that partly because we remember failed attempts at speech in the past. Bloodstein's anticipatory struggle hypothesis of stuttering is founded on that belief system. Children and adults fragment the complex task of speaking because they believe that it is necessary for them to do so in order to speak. In addition, of course, these people also remember the negative emotional arousals associated with having to speak due to failures in the past and punishment from both the listener (external) and themselves (internal). Each failure therefore reinforces the notion that speech is difficult and that fragmenting and secondary behaviours are necessary. It is a self-fulfilling and self-reinforcing paradigm. It is a paradigm based on the contributions from the amygdala-hippocampal-limbic complex that does not just make us cognitively aware of our feelings and reactions but also influences our cognitive reactions and responses, often in ways that are not in our best interests.

How we talk to ourselves about experiences and memories also reinforces, or can help modify, our belief systems. Ellis's (1984) rational emotive therapy (RET) targets just that. Rational emotive therapy challenges the belief system of the client by forcing the client and clinician to evaluate emotional consequences of events in a more rational and honest manner. Instead of reinforcing irrational beliefs ('I'll never be able to talk better!') the client learns to evaluate events realistically and more honestly – what Ellis refers to as 'more rationally'. In this way the belief system can be cognitively modified; responses that were conditioned and reinforced by an inappropriate belief system can be altered and new responses can be learned in their place.

Remember that this cognitive consideration of conditioned responses is undoubtedly known to the amygdala via the cortical connections with the frontal lobes of both hemispheres.

We are not slaves to classical conditioning, instrumental conditioning or even operant conditioning. We are able to relearn and change responses.

The hippocampus

Our old friend, the hippocampus, also plays a major role in learning. As mentioned above, in order to learn we must be able to remember. What is stored in long-term memory must first be processed by the hippocampus. This structure is not a passive contributor to this process. The hippocampus is thought by many to conduct higher level evaluations of stimuli both in terms of input and in terms of output to the amygdala. In the 1960s, Smythies considered the hippocampus to be the structure that sent an internal representational model of the external world to the rest of the limbic system for evaluation and emotional response. This is a fairly heavy responsibility as an incorrect or misconceived representation of the external world would result in an inappropriate emotional response (as when you ask someone on a date because you thought the other person was responsive to the idea and find that you are wrong). This idea also was one of the initiators of studies into limbic-hippocampal-amygdala contributions to paranoia and schizophrenia.

Returning to Brutten and Shoemaker and their classically conditioned negative emotional responses to speaking brings us also here to the hippocampus. The two-factor theory states that this emotional response is generalized through the process of higher order conditioning and stimulus generalization. Higher order conditioning is responsible for stimuli farther and farther removed from the originating stimulus being able to elicit the same response. A good example of this involves the often unfairly maligned dentist. For a fair number of the population just calling the dental office for an appointment is sufficient to cause anxiety about the visit. It is higher order conditioning that you have to thank for that response. A second conditioning paradigm used by Brutten and Shoemaker is stimulus generalization. This explains, for instance, why some children become upset in the store if they see someone in a white coat because their doctor who immunizes them also wears such a coat. These two conditioning techniques are responsible for different but somehow related stimuli in situations far removed from but in some way related to the original being able to result in the negative emotional reaction to having to speak. This is how the emotional reaction is generalized outward from the originating milieu; and this is where an important contribution from the hippocampus comes into play. Through his own work and reviews of the work of others, LeDoux (1993a, 1993b) demonstrates that it is the hippocampus that provides the amygdala with information about the context in which the original conditioning takes place. The hippocampus is critical for contextual conditioning – that is, the learning associated with the milieu in which the unconditioned/conditioned response pairing took place. It is also the hippocampus that communicates to the amygdala the current milieu in which a response is elicited. It is through this contribution by the hippocampus that Brutten and Shoemaker's explanations of generalization through higher order conditioning and stimulus generalization can best be neurophysiologically explained. It is wonderfully elegant in simplicity: those structures responsible for memory and conditioning are also those structures that are responsible for the emotional response that they are mediating.

There is a negative side to the establishment of emotional memory and emotional conditioning. According to LeDoux (1993a, 1993b) these responses are indelible. Once established, these are ours forever. The results of elicitation can be managed cognitively but to one degree or another these responses will always come forth in response to specific and contextual stimuli. Relating these data to the treatment of stuttering is disturbingly easy to any clinician or client who has attempted to teach or establish long-term generalization and maintenance of fluency. This will be discussed in a later chapter. The next question is what happens to this hippocampal–amygdala activation and response?

The basal ganglia

One thing that happens is that the elicited and contextually reinforced emotional response is communicated upstream to the structures of the basal ganglia. Until recently, due to basal ganglia/substantia nigra implications for Parkinson's disease, this area has been ascribed primarily motor responsibilities. To be sure, this is a responsibility of this area; however, we now know that these structures also have major contributions to the learning and retention of motor behaviour. It was assumed in the past that the majority of communication involving these structures ran from them to the cortex and brainstem. It is now known that there are profuse reciprocal corticobasal connections that run from the cortex to the basal ganglia. In addition, there is reciprocal communication between the basal ganglia and the limbic system. In that schema the basal ganglia are viewed as the point of first interface between the emotional centres and the voluntary movement centres of the cortex.

Connor and Abbs reviewed sensorimotor contributions of the basal ganglia as known in 1990. Earlier reports in the literature considered the basal ganglia to be essentially separate from the cortex but acting as a modulator of the pyramidal motor system. These authors report that the separation of the basal ganglia into the so-called extrapyramidal system is no longer accurate. The cortical connections to the basal ganglia terminate most often in the putamen and are reciprocal back into those same areas and other cortical areas. These cortical areas include the motor, premotor, and somatosensory areas in primates. Interestingly, afferent projections from the putamen project through the thalamus to the supplementary motor areas and then through that area to the primary motor cortex. Conner and Abbs consider the supplementary motor area to be a location where further processing of the basal ganglia input occurs before final communication with the primary motor area. The supplementary motor area activates prior to movement onset and Connor and Abbs report that disruptions in the activation order between the basal ganglia and the supplementary motor area may be the etiology of aberrant movements associated with Parkinson's disease. (In neuroimaging studies to be reviewed in the next chapter, inappropriate deactivation of the caudate nucleus is reported as occurring in the stuttering subjects. Keep this information from Connor and Abbs in mind as you read the reviews in the next few pages.)

The putamen appears to be the structure of the basal ganglia that contributes most to control of oro-facial structures in the ventromedial zone of the basal ganglia. This area would, therefore, have reciprocal connections to those areas of the supplementary motor cortex responsible for oro-facial movement.

Both the basal ganglia and supplementary motor area respond with different magnitudes of activation depending on the sensory stimuli preceding or concomitant with movement. This presents an interesting hypothesis. Stuttering is known to decrease or disappear when speech is accompanied by auditory stimuli such as rhythmic tapping, delayed auditory feedback or masking. This induced fluency could be the partial result of more appropriate activations of the basal ganglia and supplementary motor areas. Could it be that the auditory perception of dysfluent speech may disrupt these areas' sensorimotor speech control? Conversely, then, could re-establishment of that control occur when auditory input does not include stuttered speech?

Kimura (1995) reports that there is major input from the structures of the basal ganglia in the long-term learning of movements. Neurones in the striatum demonstrate changes in their activity during behavioural sensorimotor conditioning tasks. Most of these studies have focused on the activities of the tonically active neurones (TANs) in the primate striatum. Tonically active neurones are widely but not densely distributed in the caudate nucleus and putamen. (Remember that it is the putamen that contains an oro-facial centre. Bear in mind, too, that neuroimaging studies to be reviewed in detail in the next chapter point to the caudate nucleus as being inappropriately activated during stuttering.) These TANs develop responses to the classical conditioning stimuli during classical conditioning tasks. Kimura wanted to see if these responses of the TANs could be elicited after a prolonged break in the training. That is, he wanted to see if the TANs could demonstrate learning and memory for classical conditioning over time. In order to test this the experimental monkeys enjoyed four weeks off from their laboratory work; then training resumed. It was found that the TANs retained their acquired responsiveness even after this long period of no exposure to the stimuli. In fact – and this may be fairly important to our discussion here – more TANs were found to be responding after the break in training than were responding during the training. Kimura took this to mean that the conditioned responses of the TANs acquired through weeks of training were maintained in long-term memory storage. Then, after the four-week vacation, the conditioning must have been retrieved from memory.

What is particularly interesting is that even more of the TANs were responsive after the break than before. Recall LeDoux's (1993a, 1993b) warning that emotional memories and emotional responses are indelible once classical conditioning has established these in the repertoire of conditioned responses. When that information is combined with this information concerning the learning by the striatal TANs and the fact that more of these neurones respond after a rest in conditioning, it can be argued that this indelibleness is reinforced in both the emotional centres and at the level of the striatum. No wonder stuttering can be so difficult to treat.

Kimura also found that the dopamine system of the striatum exerts considerable influence on the responses of these TANs, especially as related to behavioural learning and memory. After the conditioning research described above was completed, Kimura lesioned the nigrostriatal dopamine system on one cerebral hemisphere, thus depleting this neurochemical in the putamen and caudate nucleus on one side. This reduction resulted in a significant drop in responsiveness of the TANs in those structures on that side but not in responsiveness on the unlesioned second side. The animals retained their conditioned responses on the normal side but lost them on the lesioned side. This led Kimura to postulate that the dopamine system functioned to enable the striatum to retrieve neural activity acquired in the striatum by conditioned learning. In this scheme, the dopamine system is seen as the system that modulates neural activity in the striatum during learning of sensorimotor tasks as well as in the future when the dopamine allows the TANs to retrieve and perform conditioned learning from memory stores. It is through this dopamine system that the TANs may act to influence the initiation of conditioned behaviours as well as strongly contributing to the long-term maintenance of those behaviours.

Kimura reminds us the caudate nucleus, putamen, nucleus accumbens can be divided into functional zones based on the cortical and subcortical inputs each zone receives. One such zone receives input from the sensorimotor cortex, the parietal and prefrontal association cortices, and another from the limbic system, including the anterior cingulate gyrus and the orbital cortices. Kimura suggests that the motor, cognitive and emotional systems from these areas can therefore interact within the caudate nucleus and putamen. This is particularly true of the limbic system as, compared to the cerebellum and motor cortex, the basal ganglia receive large amounts of input from the limbic system. This limbic input in particular enjoys a preferred distribution in the ventral striatum, caudate nucleus and putamen. This input reaches these structures via at least two routes. One is from the direct inputs from the amygdala, midline thalamus, and prefrontal cortex. The second is from dopamine-containing neurones in the substantia nigra pars compacta. Kimura contends that the dopamine-containing neurones of the substantia nigra compacta must be under tight control by the limbic system as it is in the limbic system where external as well as internal stimuli are evaluated.

Kimura's conclusion is that the basal ganglia may well be the area of integration between cognitive and limbic motor input. In this way the basal ganglia participate in the mechanisms of intended behaviour.

These data on the dopamine system's necessary role as a TAN activator are particularly interesting in light of a report by Wu and colleagues (1997). These researchers used positron emission tomography (PET) scans to determine increases in dopamine uptake activity in normal-speaking subjects and in subjects who stuttered. Excess dopamine levels had been previously implicated in stuttering as dopamine uptake inhibitors have been reported to decrease the frequency and severity of stuttering (Wu et al., 1995). In the 1997 study, stuttering subjects demonstrated almost three times the normal uptake of dopamine in the ventral median prefrontal cortex (the cingulate) and a greater than 100% increase in uptake in limbic structures such as the left amygdala, left insular cortex, left caudate nucleus and right deep orbital cortex. The medial prefrontal cortex, which was shown to have a threefold dopamine increase in the subjects who stuttered, is functionally connected to the supplemental motor areas. Both of these areas are known to have significant contributions to the initiation and control of vocalizations in primate and humans.

Based on Kimura's data we should not be surprised about either the increased dopamine uptake or the fact that such a huge increase in dopamine uptake was found in the caudate nucleus of the striatum as well as limbic associated areas and the left amygdala. If we apply Kimura's data to Wu's it can be hypothesized that TANs of the caudate nucleus are responding proportionally to the uptake of dopamine. This inappropriate dopamine uptake results in the TANs, especially in the ventral putamen (the oro-facial control area), over responding. This over-response of the TANs could contribute to the oro-facial speech-related behaviours associated with stuttering. The over-response is also a factor of the amygdala, which has profuse connections with both the striatum and the cortical centres for motor activity. Thus, a reciprocal cycle of over-response may be set into motion with each level from the amygdala to the striatum to the cortex and back serving to both stimulate more dopamine uptake and reinforce the over-activity that requires the dopamine increase – a perfect example of the cyclic nature of stuttering.

This chapter and the previous chapter have presented data that show the relationships among the striatum, amygdala and hippocampus that are necessary for conditioned learning to take place. Wu's data and the other studies reviewed in this and the previous chapter serve to support the hypothesis that stuttering is the result of limbic system input into the various subcortical and cortical sensorimotor areas responsible for both vocalization and verbalization. In this model, negative emotional arousal – initially manifested as a fear response – is established as a conditioned response. This conditioning is achieved through the combined contributions of emotional-limbic responses, especially those involving the hippocampus and amygdala. The cognitive component of the response emerges when the child's belief system includes the belief that, for him or her, talking is a difficult behaviour to successfully initiate and complete. Both of these learned aspects – the emotional and the cognitive – converge in the basal ganglia. One result of these learned responses is an increased uptake of dopamine, especially by the oro-facial centres in the putamen as well as centres in the caudate nucleus. The result of dopamine-induced over-response by the basal ganglia is the neurophysiologically determined tonic or clonic block at the onset of speech. As will be illustrated in the next chapter, the subcortical and cortical emotional and prosodic areas of the right hemisphere are also recipients of this inappropriate limbic-basal ganglia activation. These centres respond by contributing emotional reaction and prosodic input into dominant left hemisphere speech areas that are incompatible with fluency. The result of all this activity is stuttering. In order to prevent, overcome or escape this activity, the child learns to incorporate the secondary behaviours so closely associated with the speech behaviours of stuttering. These are temporarily effective because they serve to lessen the dopamine increase caused by the original conditioning. This increase is lessened because the new instrumental conditioning serves to temporarily dampen or inhibit a full conditioned response from being elicited by the hippocampal-amygdala-basal ganglia interface. Over time this inhibition becomes less and less effective until replaced by a new (novel) response and that cycle continues. This instrumental learning results in a chained series of behaviours, with each link in the chain serving to act as a cue for emergence of the next. Stuttering is so difficult to treat in the older client because this emotionally based learning founded on fear and negative emotional response becomes indelible. The responses can be cognitively and behaviourally dealt with but will, to one degree or another, be called up whenever the environmental constellation of stimuli is sufficiently similar to the originating stimuli and milieu. In this manner learning and neurophysiology combine – as they would have to – and result in stuttering and the individual's attempt to cope with it.

Chapter Three
Neuroimaging studies of stuttering

Now that you have the basic information about the cortical and subcortical areas and structures that seem to be involved in the production of both fluent and stuttered speech, it is time to take that information and apply it. Recent reports of neuroimaging studies involving subjects who stutter and fluent speakers provide an ideal avenue for this application of information. We will discuss several studies in the order of their publication. This chronology will be interesting from several perspectives. First, it will allow us to appreciate the increase in sophistication of technology in the area of non-invasive imaging of the central nervous system. Second, it will allow us to appreciate the criticisms of the earliest studies of this type and how later studies, because of technological advances, solved those early methodological problems. Last, this review will support the view that the explanation for the results to be addressed rests in the activities and connections of the subcortical areas and structures presented and discussed in the first chapter. Chapter Three will conclude with the presentation of the three dimensional model of stuttering. The model will be discussed in terms of the information in Chapter One and through the data and inference presented in the first section of this chapter.

Before beginning this section a word of qualification is in order. None of the studies to be reviewed is without its critics. For the most part these criticisms involve questions concerning the subjects used, the methodology employed or the conclusions drawn. Although the present discussion will not be criticized for the two reasons given above, inferences that will be made may well be open for questioning. This is good. The field of stuttering needs as much controversy as possible. Controversy breeds studies and studies breed findings and findings breed more controversy and – well, you get the point. Progress is sometimes not direct. Often a sailing manoeuvre called 'tacking' is the best way to describe the forward motion in the field of stuttering and fluency. When the winds are against you, tacking allows you to move back and forth but still steadily forward. It takes a lot longer to reach the destination but the alternative is to wait for the winds to change – and you can wait a long time for that.

Interest in a neurological explanation for stuttering can be traced back to the work of Orton and Travis. Theirs was the first formal theory of stuttering that had a definite etiological theory based in the central nervous system of people who stutter. Briefly, the theory is based on the idea of a lack of cerebral dominance for speech. Orton and Travis maintained that the normal left-hemispheric dominance for both speech and language was lacking in those who stuttered. In normal fluent speakers the dominant left instructs the right hemisphere motor areas to follow the left's instructions concerning speed, accuracy, range and strength of movement. When both hemispheres cooperated in sending the same innervation to their respective sides of the speech system, fluency resulted. If neither side was dominant for speech control both were able to send their own innervation signals. The resulting discoordinations to both halves of the muscles involved in speaking resulted in the overt manifestations of the disorder. The theory fell out of favour partly because the therapy prescribed by it – regaining left hemisphere dominance by only using the right arm and hand – did not work. Still, modifications of the theory keep returning over the years. It has now returned again, albeit in a greatly modified form that does not really resemble much of the original. Still, most imaging articles will mention Orton and Travis in the introductory section, mainly because many of them find an inappropriate right side activation during stuttering that is typically not seen during fluent speech in the subjects who stutter (SWS).

In 1980, Wood, Stump, McKeehan, Sheldon, and Proctor reported their results using single photon emission computed tomography (SPECT) for the first time in an investigation of stuttering. The study only used two SWS. The female subject stuttered as a result of a head injury. The male subject had stuttered since age four. The female subject presented some problems since hers was not a developmental stutter. Be that as it may, the results pointed the way for future studies. During the SPECT scans the subjects were evaluated during a stuttering event and then a second time after treatment with haloperidol, a central nervous system depressant. During the unmedicated segment the female subject demonstrated higher blood flow to all areas of the right hemisphere compared with the left. After administration of the haloperidol, the subject was reported to stutter less and her left hemisphere showed greater blood flow than her right for all anterior frontal regions.

The male subject who had a developmental stutter, showed lessened blood flow to Broca's area in the unmedicated condition and an increase in the right hemisphere in the frontal lobe area mirroring the location of Broca's on the left. This reversed after haloperidol treatment.

The authors took these findings to suggest that stuttering was the result of abnormal anterior frontal lobe activation involving the right hemisphere.

The results of this early study are somewhat contaminated by the small number of subjects and that the SWS presented different etiologies of the stuttering. It is interesting to note, though, that even with different etiologies their SPECT scans were similar in showing inappropriate activation strength by the right hemisphere and less activation in the left.

The use of haloperidol is also noteworthy. This is a major tranquillizer with very unpleasant side effects if used too long. Two of these side effects are germane to our discussion here. First, long-term administration of haloperidol is associated with tardive dyskinesia. This dyskinesia results in bizarre uncontrollable movements of the mouth and jaw. Second, Parkinson's disease-like symptoms have also been reported as a result of long-term use (Physicians Desk Reference, 1996). Both of these reactions make sense as the basal ganglia are very much targeted by this medication. Both side effects, tardive dyskinesia and Parkinson's disease, are also the result of basal ganglia disorders. As we know from the first and second chapters, the basal ganglia are very much involved in speech motor control and conditioning paradigms. The haloperidol could certainly act to depress the manifestations of conditioning associated with stuttering in the basal ganglia on the right as well as on the left and therefore result in a fluency increase.

You may be thinking that etiologies of both the above disorders include problems involving dopamine and you would be correct. Haloperidol is a dopamine blocker. It inhibits the uptake of that neurotransmitter. Increases in dopamine levels have been implicated in stuttering by Wu and associates (1997) in a study to be reviewed later in this section. By reducing the dopamine uptake the haloperidol may have reduced the effects of conditioning involving the basal ganglia via the amygdala.

Remember the TANS conditioned responses reviewed in the previous chapter and the relationship to dopamine uptakes. This reduction of the conditioned response due to inhibition by the haloperidol of dopamine uptake may have been the reason for lessened stuttering and more appropriate left hemisphere activations for speech.

This study is also noteworthy from the standpoint of the authors' suggestion that stuttering is the result of activities of the anterior cortices, especially the inappropriate activation of the right anterior frontal cortex in areas that mirror the location of Broca's area on the left. As you remember, that area on the right has been called the anterior area of Ross and is responsible for the prosodic suprasegmental inputs into ongoing sensorimotor speech. Damage results in a persistent monotone without emotional expression, regardless of the verbalization. This is an area with heavy limbic input. The anterior area of Ross translates that emotionality from the limbic areas into the emotionally laden prosody that carries so much meaning and expression in our speech. In a model that credits those limbic sites as initiators of the conditioning that ultimately results in stuttering, limbic-based overactivation of the anterior area of Ross coupled with hypoactivation of Broca's area on the left comes as no surprise. This is exactly what such a model would predict.

In 1991, Pool, Devous, Freeman, Watson, and Finitzo reported their findings using SPECT. This study investigated the regional cerebral blood flow (rCBF) in a much larger sample than Wood et al. Pool et al. used 20 SWS in their study. All subjects were evaluated for stuttering and were assigned severity classifications of mild, moderate, or severe. In addition, magnetic resonance imaging (MRI) was conducted to exclude any subject with obvious brain pathologies. All subjects passed the MRI. The SPECT evaluations of rCBF were conducted with the subjects quiet and resting. All results were significant but not without controversy as you will see.

Results of the study indicated 'global, absolute flow reductions' (p. 509) on the left hemisphere relative to the right. The authors reported that three hemispheric areas demonstrated right hemisphere increases relative to the left. These were the anterior cingulate gyrus and the superior and middle temporal gyri. There was a correlation between severity of the stuttering and rCBF results. Those diagnosed as 'severe' had large rCBF increases in the right anterior cingulate gyrus and a corresponding decrease in the left. Those diagnosed as 'mild' had a greater left rCBF in the anterior cingulate gyrus than those subjects diagnosed as either 'severe' or 'moderate'. Those diagnosed as 'moderate' had rCBF to their right anterior cingulate gyrus that fell somewhere between the values recorded for the mild and severe groups. Therefore, stuttering severity was seen to increase as a function of increased right anterior cingulate gyrus activity.

The anterior cingulate gyrus is a major contributor to speech initiation (remember the poor man with the lesion who lost the drive to speak unless he was asked to repeat verbally and then he would speak – otherwise he was silent). The cingulate gyrus also receives major input from subcortical limbic structures directly as well as through the anterior nuclei of the thalamus. Therefore, more intense conditioned limbic input would lead us to expect larger right-sided anterior cingulate gyrus activation in subjects with a severe stutter.

How are the activations of the superior and medial temporal lobes explained? First because the subjects are listening to any ambient noise. Remember, too, though, that the amygdalas are located in the mesial temporal lobes and that each amygdala has extensive connections to its respective auditory cortex. If conditioned responses from the amygdala do contribute to stuttering then one would expect at least the mesial temporal lobes to be activated partly by amygdala activation and partly by temporal lobe auditory inputs being produced into the amygdalas.

All of the above data were recorded while the SWS were silent. This methodology presents some interpretation difficulties. The authors concluded that the data strongly suggested that stuttering was the result of fundamental differences in the brain activities of those who stutter. In 1996, Ingham, Fox, Ingham and associates investigated the resting state rCBF using PET scans of 10 male SWS. This study reported no differences in rCBF values between the SWS and the normal controls.

An interesting study was conducted by Szelag et al. (1993) to evaluate the relationship between degree of right hemisphere lateralization for speech tasks and severity of stuttering in children aged 14 to 16 years' old. Nine of the SWS were classified as severe, eleven were classified as mild and there were 48 fluent control subjects. The most interesting findings were that the SWS mildly evidenced lateralizations that closely resembled the normal speaking controls. The SWS severely had significantly larger values of right hemisphere activations for all verbal and word identification tasks. The authors concluded that degree of lateralization was significantly correlated with severity of stuttering.

This was the only lateralization study using children that was found for this text. The task was a visual perception paradigm that allowed the researchers to determine which hemisphere was processing the visually presented linguistic stimuli. The use of minors for scanning studies is certainly problematic but the results would also be important. This importance should be remembered when the study by Wu and associates (1995) is reviewed as those authors suggest a specific area of persistent neurophysiological difference for SWS. If such a difference could be demonstrated in children at risk for stuttering, an objective identification method could be the result. This could result in earlier treatment and perhaps avoidance of the conditioned learning that can result in stuttering.

Ingham, Fox, and Ingham had also presented positron emission tomography results in a 1994 report. Their methodology differed substantially from earlier studies. Instead of examining their SWS while silent, these researchers examined the SWS while they were resting silently, reading aloud, and during a fluency-inducing choral reading activity. This was published as a preliminary study and had only four SWS and four control subjects.

However, this study of SWS while speaking had fascinating results. All the SWS stuttered during the reading aloud task; none stuttered during the choral activity. Results implicated the supplementary motor cortical area and the lateral premotor cortex. Whereas all activations were normal for the control group, these areas showed inappropriate activations during the reading aloud task for the SWS. During that task the supplementary motor areas of the SWS were activated more on the left than the right, while their premotor cortices were more activated on the right than the left. These abnormalities resolved during the fluency-induced choral reading task.

Recall that the brain controls the body in a contralateral fashion. The right hemisphere is responsible for the left side of the body and the left hemisphere is responsible for the right. The above results suggest that stuttering may be due to a lack of co-ordination between two cortical areas with heavy motor speech responsibilities.

It is interesting to note that during stuttering the left supplementary motor area was activated more than the right. This makes sense. The supplementary motor area of the dominant left side acts as a functional bridge between the anterior area of Ross, which is responsible for prosody and is located on the right anterior frontal lobe and Broca's area on the left. The 1980 study by Wood et al. showed increased rCBF to the anterior area of the right frontal lobe in SWS – couple these findings with left supplementary motor area over-activation and a hypothesis emerges. The hypothesis would be that, as the left supplementary motor area acts as a bridge between the prosodic centre on the right and Broca's area on the left, over-activation of the left supplementary motor area would indicate that it is forwarding inappropriately high input from the anterior area of Ross into Broca's area. This inappropriate input may result in an inability of Broca's area to co-ordinate its responsibilities for motor speech with those of the prosodic centre on the right. As you will see in the studies below, hypoactivation of Broca's area during stuttering will be an important finding.

In addition, Goldberg's (1985) model, which presents the supplementary motor area as an evolutionary extension of the limbic system, is worth considering here. If this is a tenable hypothesis, it also helps to explain why the left supplementary motor area was more activated than the right. Goldberg considers the supplementary motor area to depend at the subcortical level on the basal ganglia. He also views the cortical area as the intermediary between the drive-controlling mechanisms of the cingulate gyrus and the selection and execution of specific movements or strategies of movements. Moreover, Goldberg considers the supplementary motor area to be part of the cortico-limbic-reticular system and in that role it serves to direct limbic input into motor areas, in this case into Broca's area.

The left supplementary motor area would, therefore, be overactivated because the task being mediated is speech, a motor function of the dominant left hemisphere. The left supplementary motor area is acting as a bridge for the confluence of inputs from the right-sided anterior area of Ross, from the basal ganglia, and from the limbic system. It is then feeding that information into the primary motor areas as well as into Broca's area. The supplementary motor area of the left hemisphere would therefore be the logical choice to display increased rCBF during stuttering.

In 1995, Wu, Maguire, Riley and colleagues used PET scans to investigate the brain functioning of four SWS while fluent and when stuttering. Four fluent control subjects were also included. The scans were obtained while the SWS read aloud to another person and when they were engaged in a fluency-inducing choral reading activity. Several really interesting results were obtained. First, Wu et al. think that they may have identified a trait marker for stuttering. The concepts of trait and state need some explanation here. It is easiest to explain these two through the perspective of anxiety. Trait anxiety is the level of anxiety that we carry around with us all the time. Some of us are more anxious than others and one can say that those people have a higher trait anxiety than those who are less anxious all the time. State anxiety is anxiety created by circumstances; it sums with the trait anxiety. Put people with high trait anxiety in an anxiety-producing circumstance and their resulting anxiety level is higher than someone with low trait anxiety in the same circumstance. Wu and his associates think that they have discovered a neurophysiological trait marker for people who stutter. That is, they think that this trait marker is there all the time, whether the person who stutters is fluent or stuttering. Their results show a 50% lower activity level for the left caudate nucleus in their SWS – whether those subjects are stuttering or fluent.

In addition to that finding, they also found a reversible hypoactivity of Broca's area and, interestingly, of Wernicke's area during stuttering; reduced activity in the bilateral superior frontal lobe higher association areas, the right cerebellum, the left deep frontal orbital limbic areas, and the bilateral posterior cingulate areas. None of the SWS demonstrated greater neural activity during stuttering than during fluency; only reduced activity of the scanned regions of interest.

Let us discuss the possible trait marker of permanent hypoactivity in the left caudate nucleus last and begin with the finding of reversible hypoactivity in Broca's and Wernicke's areas. The hypoactivity of Broca's area makes perfect sense. While the SWS were stuttering, they no longer had voluntary control over their speech system, especially the articulatory portion.

This voluntary control is lost because Broca's area is no longer able to allow them that voluntary control. It is surprising that no hyperactivity was found in any area of interest during stuttering, especially in the cingulate and limbic areas. In this finding, the Wu et al. results stand alone.

Under-activation of Wernicke's area during stuttering is also understandable. This is the cortical seat of auditory verbal processing. The key word here is 'verbal'. The repetitions and tonic positioning of stuttering blocks may simply not be identified as verbalizations. Instead, those stuttered attempts at verbalization might be identified by auditory areas below Wernicke's as vocalizations, not meaningful word-production attempts.

Under-activation of the bilateral superior frontal lobe higher association areas may be due to the involuntary nature of stuttering. These four subjects were classified as having severe stutters. After all, what higher level associations could be going on during severe blocks? The SWS is locked in a muscular contest within him or herself, not an intellectual one.

During stuttering, the limbic areas – the deep frontal orbital areas and posterior cingulate areas – were underactivated. Only during the fluency-induced condition were these areas over-activated. Wu and associates do not really offer a good explanation for this effect. They only state the stuttering is associated with increased anxiety, hardly a satisfying statement in light of their findings. However, one should remember that the fear of stuttering occurs before the act of stuttering. Once the stuttering happens there is nothing to be feared; the feared activity has occurred. It was only during fluency when Wu's SWS were concerned about the possibility of stuttering that their limbic areas were activated. The concern of those SWS could have centred on their anxiety about how long they could maintain their fluency and thus the limbic activity during fluent reading activities.

What about this trait marker that may have been found in the persistent 50% less activity in the left caudate nucleus of the SWS whether stuttering or fluent? This is very curious. We should remember, and Wu points out, that only four SWS were used. In addition, Wu clearly indicates that the four controls were poorly matched in terms of age. Still, any indication of a trait marker creates speculation about whether Wu has found the heredi- tary marker for stuttering.

We have known both anecdotally and statistically that stuttering runs in families. Kidd (1984) presented evidence of a hereditary component to the disorder. What was interesting was that the report of Kidd bridged the nature/nurture argument about behaviour and heredity. Kidd suggested that the predisposition to stutter was handed down. The environment had to somehow pull the trigger that would result in the predisposition becoming reality. The left caudate nucleus in the SWS may represent the genetically deficient central nervous system structure that is vulnerable to environmental triggering. If a child is born with a left caudate that is only functioning at a 50% level then it may be the weak link in the speech production system that is under such pressure as the child acquires speech and language skills. Such a weak link might allow the acquisition of conditioned fear responses that result in dysfluency to be learned more easily than the child with no family history of stuttering and with a fully operating caudate nucleus. Such a child would be at lower risk for stuttering because there would be no subcortical motor speech controller with compromised functioning.

Last, Wu and colleagues also reported that, during fluency, the SWS had an over-activated substantia nigra. This area is concerned with the produc- tion of dopamine. Death of this area results in Parkinson's disease due to lack of sufficient dopamine for use by the basal ganglia. This too is a curious finding, especially in light of a later report by Wu et al. (1997) that demonstrates increased levels of dopamine to be associated with increased severity of stuttering.

The above findings stand alone in reports of imaging studies of stuttering. As indicated earlier, the SWS used in the study were older than the controls and were classified as severe. The age range of the SWS was between 20 and 54 with a mean age of nearly 42 years. The controls' age range was between 22 and 41 years with a mean of 30 years. All of the previously discussed results and the studies left to be presented used younger SWS. Whether this is significant is currently a matter for conjecture; however, the age of the SWS and the small number of them – four – could both result in unusual findings. Couple those problems with the fact that there are probably subgroups of people who stutter – people who stutter due to differing values of central nervous system and environmental variables – and it becomes easier to understand sometimes anomalous findings in the field of stuttering and fluency, even in studies as objective as neuroimaging.

Fox, Ingham, Ingham and associates (1996) found just the opposite of the Wu et al. results discussed above. The Fox et al. study used PET scans to investigate neural activities in controls and SWS when fluent and during stuttering. These authors report that the stuttering resulted in widespread over-activations of the cerebral and cerebellar motor systems with a clear right hemisphere dominance.

During stuttering, the SWS evidenced over-activations of the mouth area of the primary motor strip on the right, significantly larger activations of the supplementary motor areas, strong activations of the superior lateral premotor cortex, and cerebellar activations more than double those in the fluent controls. Activations seen only in the SWS included the bilateral insulas, the claustrum, globus pallidus, and lateral thalamus, all on the left side. Activation of the left superior temporal lobes, seen in the normal controls, was absent in the SWS. This temporal gyrus is active during vocalized self-monitoring activities. (These auditory cortices were not activated in the SWS in the Wu et al. results reviewed above either.)

Areas that were normally activated during a choral fluency-inducing activity in the SWS were also found to be deactivated during the stuttering. These were the left inferior frontal cortex (Brodman's area 47) and the superior and posterior temporal cortices (Brodman's area 22). The posterior area of the temporal lobe, area 22, is, of course, Wernicke's area.

During the choral reading induced-fluency task most of the above abnormal activations or deactivations reversed and the SWS resembled the normal controls. This was true except for activations of the supplementary motor areas and mouth area of the primary motor strip. Both of these remained right hemisphere dominant in activation strength.

Based on these results the authors concluded that stuttering was the result of a dysfunctional fronto-temporal system for verbal fluency. These results were very consistent across the stuttering severity range in the SWS. The same activations or deactivations were observed regardless of the severity classification assigned to the individual SWS. (This finding does not agree with Szelag et al. (1993) reviewed above, but then she and her associates used a visual perception task to assess hemispheric dominance, not neuroimaging.) Fox et al. conclude by stating that their results support several theories of stuttering but that what is needed is a unifying theory that is of enough scope to include the complex actions and interactions observed in their work as well as in the work of others. Seems reasonable.

Table 3.1: Results of imaging studies

Authors	Number of Subjects	Image	Results
Wood et al., 1980	2	SPECT	Increased blood flow to right hemisphere. Decreased blood flow to Broca's area. Increased blood flow to frontal lobe on right.
Pool et al., 1991	20	SPECT	Global blood flow decrease on left hemisphere. Blood flow increase on right hemisphere. r: between blood flow and stuttering severity.
Szelag et al., 1993	20	Visual perception	Right hemisphere activations. r: between severity and amount of activation.
Ingham et al., 1994	4	PET	Activation of S.M.A. on left, lateral premotor cortex on right.
Wu et al., 1995	4	PET	Decreased activation of left caudate nucleus. Decreased activation of Broca's and Wernicke's areas. Bilateral reduced activity of superior frontal lobes. Reduced activity of right cerebellum, left deep orbital limbic areas and bilateral posterior cingulate areas.
Fox et al., 1996	10	PET	Increased activation of primary motor strip for the mouth, SMAS, superior lateral premotor cortex, cerebellum, bilateral insulas, claustrum, globus pallidus and the lateral left thalamus.

The above results implicate both cortical and subcortical areas and structures in stuttering. As in the Wu et al. results above, these findings were consistent regardless of whether the SWS were stuttering or fluent. Wu and associates found the severe underactivation of the caudate nucleus on the left, whereas Fox et al. found right-hemisphere dominance for the supplementary motor area and the mouth area on the primary motor strip. Both of these sets of researchers also found abnormal activations of the basal ganglia structures – Wu et al. of the caudate and Fox et al. of the claustrum and globus pallidus. Kimura (1995) considers the basal ganglia to be the area of interface between the limbic system and the motor system in the human brain – the point at which emotionality affects motor performance. With that in mind, it comes as no surprise that the structures of the basal ganglia are implicated by two separate studies in the disorder of stuttering.

The right side supplementary motor area was consistently activated in the SWS regardless of the verbal condition. This is interesting as well. It does not agree with Wu et al., above, who found left-side activations of that area in their SWS. Be that as it may, overactivation or underactivation of either side during speech may be considered an abnormal function as it would indicate a lack of hemispheric co-ordination of innervation to speech musculature. Overactivation of the supplementary motor area on the right suggests that limbic inputs from right-sided limbic structures are occurring. As you may remember, Goldberg (1985) postulated that the supplementary motor areas are evolutionary extensions of the limbic system and have heavy limbic input. In addition, the supplementary motor areas have subcortical dependence on the basal ganglia, two structures of which were abnormally activated during the stuttering condition in the SWS. The fact that these were on the left side makes sense since speech is a left hemispheric function; therefore, those left-side structures supporting speech would be activated. The right-side supplementary motor area was activated due to heavy right-side limbic input that was communicated to subcortical speech controllers on the left via the corpus callosum and other smaller subcortical commissural tracts.

What of the cerebellum activations that were more than doubled in the SWS compared to the fluently speaking controls? As presented in Chapter One, there is a growing body of evidence implicating the cerebellum in higher-level brain functions in addition to the responsibilities of motor control traditionally assigned to it. Two of these higher-level functions are important here. One is cerebellar contributions to speech and language; the other is cerebellar contributions and responses to emotional expression. Via the hypothalamus, the lateral aspect of the cerebellum, the neocerebellum, has direct reciprocal connections with the hypothalamus. The hypothalamus is a major source of output of limbic responses. One route by which emotionality that is associated with speaking and stuttering may be communicated from the limbic area to Broca's area and other speech motor areas in the frontal lobe is through the neocere-bellum. The neocerebellum connects with the motor and speech areas of the frontal lobes through the ventrolateral and central lateral nuclei of the thalamus. Although an initial explanation for the level of cerebellar activation being doubled in the SWS might be that this area is involved in attempting to establish coordination of the uncoordinated articulators, an expanded explanation would include the cerebellar inputs into the frontal lobe speech motor areas of limbic input as well as cerebellar influence in both speech and language.

This cognitive/language influence has been discussed earlier. Suffice it to say here that the neocerebellum is considered to be a functional area that acts as a bridge between Broca's and Wernicke's areas as well as being involved in actual language abilities such as naming. With this information in mind it is easier to understand and appreciate why there would be double the cerebellar activation during stuttering in the SWS.

In 1997, Wu, Maguire, Riley and associates published their PET scan data indicating that stuttering was associated with increased dopamine activity. Three SWS were compared with six fluent subjects. The SWS were free of any medical complications and were taking no medication at the time of the study. They were classified as having a moderate or severe stutter. Wu and colleagues stated that, as far as they knew, this was the first report of dopamine uptake differences between SWS and fluent controls. (There is at least one earlier report of increased dopamine production associated with stuttering. This was a non-English publication reported by Lastovka (1995). The results from Chimelova (1975) indicated a 400% increase in production of adrenaline, a 300% increase in noradrenaline and a 200% increase in dopamine after SWS spoke and stuttered for 30 to 60 minutes.) Remember that dopamine uptake is associated with decreased cerebral activity. A previous report by Wu et. al. (1995) associated decreased activation of the cerebrum with a decrease in stuttering.

These authors reported three times the uptake of dopamine in the SWS compared to fluent controls. One assumes that this occurred during silence as no speaking or stuttering was reported as part of the methodology. This increased uptake was seen in the right ventral medial prefrontal cortex and the left tail of the caudate nucleus. Compared with the controls the SWS demonstrated a greater than 100% increase in limbic structures such as the extended amygdala, left insular cortex, and right deep orbital cortex. In their 1995 study, Wu and associates also identified the ventral cortical regions as being involved in a circuit for stuttering. The medial prefrontal cortex is functionally connected to the supplementary motor areas on both hemispheres. Remember, that the supplementary motor areas are considered by Penfield (1959) and by Wu et al. (!997) to be the vocalization centre in primates. Penfield went so far as to call it the third speech centre.

Wu et al. concluded that results concerning the limbic cortical areas suggested that mesodopamine tracks could be inappropriately overactive in the SWS. Wu and his colleagues do qualify the results due to the small sample size.

How can it be that researchers such as Fox et al. (1996) and the Wu study find such different results? Fox reported overactivation of some areas that Wu reports as being underactivated, as suggested by high dopamine uptake. Wu and associates also find stuttering to be reduced when dopamine blockers are administered (1995). Well, first, it does not appear that the SWS were speaking when the blood samples and PET scans were taken. Second, it may well be that these areas identified by Wu et al. are in fact underactivated during silence and overactivated during speech and stuttering. It could also be that one outcome of conditioning associated with stuttering is abnormal dopamine uptake by the brain structures and areas involved either in the conditioning or as part of the conditioned response. Recall the results of Kimura (1995) and the effects of dopamine on TAN memory and learning. What is notable from our standpoint here is the same structures named as crucial to conditioning (the amygdala and those of the basal ganglia), and vocalization and verbalization (the cerebellum, anterior cingulate gyrus and supplementary motor areas) are seen again as structures and areas involved in stuttering. One hopes that future research will unravel the seemingly disparate findings represented by both of the Wu reports (1995, 1997) in comparison with the other reports reviewed in this chapter. One wishes that Wu and associates would have discussed such differences in both of their articles.

In summary, this chapter has reviewed the most current imaging studies involving stuttering. For the most part these studies indicate overactivation of structures and areas discussed in Chapters One and Two as contributing to the emotional, motoric and learning aspects of developmental stuttering. These same areas and structures are referred to in these articles: the amygdala, the basal ganglia, the cerebellum, the frontal motor speech areas and the auditory areas of the temporal lobe.

Not every study reviewed found the same areas/structures activated (or underactivated). This could be because of differing methodologies, probable subject differences, different regions of interest as well as the fact that there may well be subgroups in stuttering that make for a heterogeneous population in terms of etiologies and effects of learning on associated brain areas. What is consistent, however, is the similarity between subcortical, thalamic, cerebellar and cortical areas considered by this text to be involved in both the establishment, expression, and maintenance of stuttering and the results of the most current imaging studies.

Before ending this chapter, this seems to be a good place to attend to the question of so-called non-emotional stuttering that is often raised by my behaviourist-oriented friends. If stuttering has its roots in emotional centres of the brain, as suggested here, how can it be that people who stutter report stuttering in the absence of any internal emotional arousal – positive or negative? One answer may be found in the similar concepts of kindling and long-term potentiation of responses. Kindling is a technique that has been used to investigate seizure activity in experimental animals. Briefly, it consists of repeatedly stimulating temporal areas with a low electrical charge. Seizures can then be triggered with less stimulation and are then observed to spread along the sites of the kindled areas (Gloor, 1997).

This technique reveals those researchers' view that kindling exemplifies abnormal activity within the brain. On the other side of this fence are those who view kindling as the neural mechanism responsible for memory formations, the ability to recall memories and as a naturally occurring neural phenomenon that enhances both learning as well as limbic responses. These enhanced limbic responses are always manifested as hyper responses – the kindled response is exaggerated and greater than the same response prior to kindling. Kindled limbic responses are also much easier to elicit than new, just-acquired limbic responses (Gloor, 1997; Adamec, in Livingston, 1976).

These experimental results can also be viewed from the perspective of non-emotional stuttering. If, and this is controversial in the kindling research world, kindling can serve as a model for memory establishment and learning, then it may help to explain non-emotional stuttering. In fact, Van Riper (in Ham, 1986) may have inadvertently been addressing this phenomenon through his stuttering therapy. Non-emotional stuttering may be the result of kindled circuits linking the limbic, cerebellar, thalamic and basal ganglia to motor areas of the cortex. An adult who stutters may not have to experience the degree of arousal associated with development of the conditioned responses when a child. As a young child in the acquisition stage of developmental stuttering, the autonomic arousals resulting from conditioned fear responses to speaking may be significantly high. In that same adult, kindling theory would explain why the motor responses would be kindled but not necessarily the autonomic responses. The autonomic responses could lessen whereas the kindled circuits to frontal motor areas could strengthen. Remember that according to LeDoux (1993b) emotional memory and conditioning is indelible. Autonomic responses to those memories lessen. However, repeated daily activation of inappropriate motor responses may kindle those motor circuits and result in greater strength of response on that end of the process.

Another possible explanation may be found in long-term potentiation (LTP) studies. This is a phenomenon closely associated with the kindling concept. Long-term potentiation refers to continued discharge after the stimulus is stopped. It also results in augmentation of that response over time (Gloor, 1997). It is considered by some to represent the neural substrate of learning and memory (Gloor, 1997). LTP is an exciting concept to neuroscientists because it is an electrophysiological condition that can be studied through *in vivo* slices of such structures as the hippocampus. Gloor (1997) reviews such studies. He tells us that, after very small electrical stimulation of live slices of hippocampal tissue, the response from activated areas is augmented by a single charge and that the neural response in the hippocampal cells increases the probability of an action potential discharge from those same cells. In this way motor areas subjected to LTP from limbic, cerebellar, and basal ganglia areas may activate more easily and with more strength over time. Depending on the environment, autonomic arousal may or may not accompany such activation, and the result could be non-emotional stuttering.

Van Riper (in Ham, 1986) may have addressed both the concepts of kindling and LTP in his cancellation phase of stuttering therapy. In this phase the client is required to stutter through the dysfluent word then cancel it by relaxing the articulators. The client then stutters again on that word using a controlled voluntary dysfluency different from the original true dysfluency. Van Riper thought that one benefit from this technique would be to weaken the conditioned neural pathways responsible for the original involuntary stutter. In other words, the client was hopefully establishing competing LTP and kindling appropriate neural pathways that are responsible for more normal fluency.

While we are addressing our behaviourist friends, this would also be a good place to discuss how a behaviour as punishing as stuttering is maintained over time. Punishing a behaviour is the quickest way to extinguish that behaviour. Stuttering is punished by the internal reactions to it and by some rude and thoughtless listener reactions. How can it be maintained? Behavioural theory would explain this through paradigms involving the timing of positive reinforcement of tension reduction, for instance, which occurs prior to the punishment, thus maintaining the behaviour.

The above reviews suggest an alternative explanation. Stuttering is maintained because the originating sources of the conditioned responses that result in stuttering are located in emotional centres of the limbic, thalamic, cerebellar and basal ganglia areas. This original response learning is indelible – it is with the person to one degree or another forever. The strength of the emotional response may vary with the environmental stimuli that trigger it but it remains in the face of positive, negative, or punishing responses from within or without. Oddly enough, a statement about opera can exemplify this concept: if you love opera from the first time you hear it, you'll love opera forever. If you don't like it the first time, you can learn to like it; but you will never love it as much as the person who loved it when it was first heard. Your emotional reaction just will not match his or hers. You can modify emotional responses to opera or to speaking, but you cannot eradicate them. So, non-emotional stuttering and maintenance of a punished behaviour occur – and so does your reaction to Puccini.

The limbic model

Figures 3.1 to 3.7 illustrate the limbic model. In the interest of avoiding using just less than the total number of arrows fired at Custer's last stand

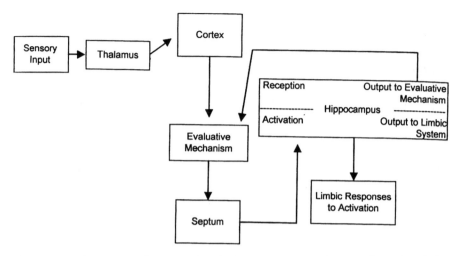

Figure 3.1: The proposed process by which incoming stimuli are evaluated and elicit limbic activation.

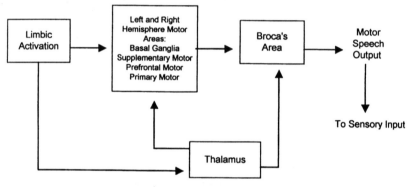

Figure 3.2: Limbic activation inputs into Broca's area via motor areas and the thalamus.

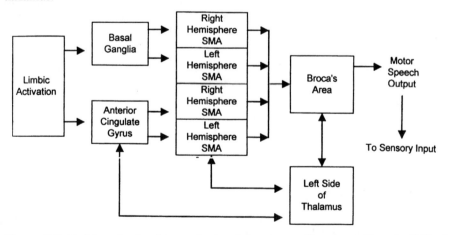

Figure 3.3: Limbic activation inputs via cingulate gyrus and basal ganglia to the SMA of both hemispheres and Broca's area via the left side of the thalamus.

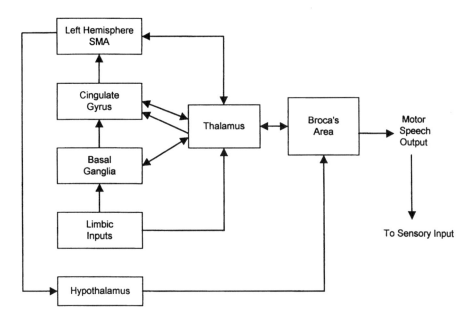

Figure 3.4: Limbic inputs to SMA via the cingulate gyrus and basal ganglia; inputs of these structures to the thalamus.

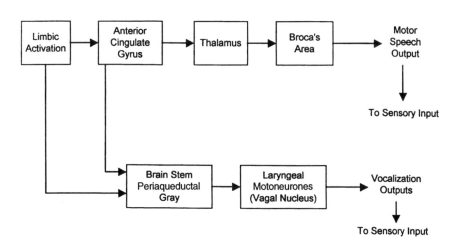

Figure 3.5: Limbic output via the anterior cingulate gyrus to Broca's area and the laryngeal motoneurones.

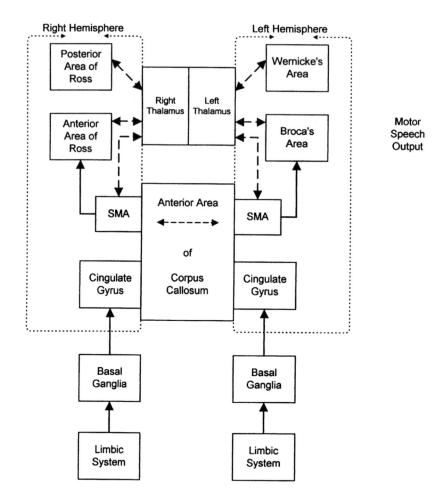

Figure 3.6: Input routes of right hemisphere areas of Ross into Broca's area.

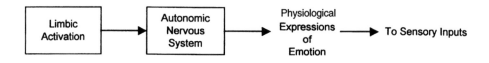

Figure 3.7: Limbic input to autonomic nervous system.

(or, for those of you in England, at Gordon's) single arrows have been used. Basically, the model states the following:

1. Incoming environmental stimuli are evaluated by the limbic system for emotional reaction. Over time a conditioned fear reaction to speaking is established by the limbic system and basal ganglia. The exact nature of the environmental stimuli that result in fear may be individualized. The reaction may be augmented by vulnerable basal ganglia especially in the male, since there is preliminary evidence from Wu et al. (1995) suggesting an underactivated caudate nucleus as a trait marker in SWS.
2. This emotional response is transmitted to the basal ganglia and cerebellum. Responses at those points are transmitted to laryngeal motor neurones and the periaqueductal grey of the midbrain and to frontal lobe motor areas, including the cingulate gyrus and prosodic motor area on the right. These inputs may result in overactivations and learning associated with long-term potentiation and the kindling phenomenon. Due to a predominant overactivation of right hemisphere areas due to limbic and basal ganglia input there is a lessening of left hemisphere dominance over motor speech planning and initiation.
3. The results of these inputs are the characteristic tonic and clonic blocks that characterize stuttering.
4. The individual attempts to compensate through struggle and secondary behaviours. The secondary behaviours, especially, are seen as instrumental behaviours, each of which over time comes to be chained to the next. These behaviours then act as cues for continuation of the inappropriate motor responses that result from the conditioned fear response and a learned cycle is begun.
5. This learned limbic-originated fear response is indelible. It may be modified by time and/or treatment but remains as a part of the individual's repertoire of learned emotional responses to the environment.
6. Fear and continued experiences with fluency failure shape the individual's belief system. Individuals come to consider themselves as 'stutterers' and to believe that speaking is, for them, a difficult and fearful activity. Each fluency failure reinforces those beliefs and a terrible cycle is born that acts to reinforce and feed itself.

This is not a model without hope. Treatment, especially early treatment in the case of children, can be very effective but, since the problem of stuttering results from a variety of contributions, each of those contributors must be addressed in the treatment. As will be explained in Chapter Four, this treatment must not only modify the overt behaviours but must also address the individual's belief system. The belief system is a cognitive correlate of the limbic system. What we believe is based not just on what we have experienced but also on our emotional reactions to those experi-

ences. Treating only the behaviour is addressing only half the package –
what that client believes about himself or herself and what is believed
about speaking must also be addressed. If not, behavioural change
cannot be maintained because there is no accompanying basic emotional
change in their beliefs or to speech. This results in the eventual re-
emergence of the stuttering because the emotional dimension of the
disorder has not been addressed.

Chapter Four
Diagnostics

The preceding information is interesting from a 'cause of symptom' perspective. We know a great deal about what is happening within the central nervous system during a stuttering event. We have yet to determine a single etiology for those central nervous system responses. This is strange from a 'diagnostic and treatment' perspective. There are not many disorders that can lay claim to being diagnosed and treated without the benefit of knowing the etiology of the problem. Stuttering can be diagnosed and successfully treated using a variety of instruments and techniques. The information and theory in this text suggest that stuttering arises and is maintained from neurology, behaviour, and emotion. One does not need an MRI or PET scan to diagnose stuttering and, certainly, neither will have any effect on treatment. Surgery is no answer – despite what some have said concerning the basal ganglia. (There has been some talk of performing stereotaxic surgery for stuttering in much the same way that the procedure is used to treat Parkinson's disease.) The neurological view is an explanation, not an option. Stuttering is certainly behaviour with emotional ramifications in terms of etiology, maintenance, diagnosis and treatment. It is, therefore, from the standpoint of behaviour and emotion that we will discuss diagnosis and treatment. Keep in mind, though, that, if successful, the treatment has to result in some neurological change, probably on a neurotransmitter, biochemical level.

The information presented in the previous chapters has definite implications for both diagnosis and treatment. Traditional diagnostic testing for stuttering is concerned with answering two primary questions. The first question is, in the case of a child, whether the child stutters or whether the dysfluency is of a normal type characterized by an excessive number of so-called normal dysfluencies. If so, then one may more confidently aim to increase fluency as opposed to decreasing stuttering. The second question, for both children and adults diagnosed as stuttering, has to do with the severity of the stuttering and the predominant type of block, the presence of struggle and/or secondary behaviours and the determination of the best therapy to address all of that. In addition, some therapists may make a judgement concerning whether or not formal emotional counselling is called for or whether they as therapists should include light counselling as part of the formal treatment package. Let us discuss each of these components through what we know about the neurophysiology of stuttering. This makes sense because, ultimately, any treatment technique is successful or not depending on whether it has been able to alter, inhibit, or increase neurological events related to sensorimotor speech initiation and control.

Is the child stuttering?

This gives rise to the issue of the importance of the distinction between dysfluencies that are 'normal' and 'not normal', especially when the number is the question. A more important question than that is 'what is the child's reaction to the dysfluencies – "normal" or not?' If the child is concerned, or if the parents are concerned, then the child and the parents should be enrolled in therapy whether or not any struggle or secondary behaviours are present. The obvious reason for this is because we want to protect the child's belief system. Conditioning of limbic and basal ganglia structures is a consequence to be avoided at all cost due to the seeming permanence of such learning. When cognitive and emotional reactions to the act of speaking begin to reinforce one another the chances for successful fluency begin to deteriorate exponentially.

If the child is stuttering then it is of utmost importance to evaluate the emotional reactions to the stutter. The emotional reactions will be there, even if not overt and obvious. My advice is not to treat the head and hope that the heart will follow; that is, don't expect to change the emotions because you change the overt behaviour. The point of this whole exercise, after all, is to convince you that stuttering is a disorder that originates from three sources – neurology, behaviour and emotion – and therefore also to convince you that diagnosis and treatment must address all three of those parameters to best serve the client who stutters. The fact that all three originate from common areas and structures should underscore the rationale that for the treatment to be as successful as possible all three components of the disorder must be addressed both diagnostically and therapeutically.

How does one evaluate the neurological aspects of the disorder? If one has unlimited funds and interest in the process, one could order neuroimaging to determine if there is characteristic overactivation of the caudate nucleus, as suggested in the previous chapter. In lieu of this, the neurological aspect can be assessed through the behavioural and emotional aspects. Both arise from the child's nervous system and the stuttering aspects arise from specific areas and structures along with the emotional aspects. First comes the emotional reaction to speaking, then comes the conditioning, then the tonic and/or clonic stuttering blocks and last come the struggle and secondary behaviours.

Assessing the emotional reaction can be as easy as asking the parents, the child or the teachers. Observation of the child in the classroom as well as observation of the classmates when the child is verbalizing can be of great help. Struggle behaviour is an indicator of emotional involvement. It shows the frustration and the involuntary nature of the dysfluencies. Secondary behaviours are also positive for emotional reaction. These show that the child wishes to avoid, lessen, or escape the dysfluency because of the negative emotional reactions, both internal and external, associated with the blocks.

Diagnostically assessing the behaviours of stuttering in children is not easy. One can do frequency counts of syllables or words stuttered per minute, how these were stuttered, and whether or not struggle or secondary behaviours were evidenced. Students are typically taught that these are 'objective' methods that are somehow superior to 'subjective' methods – i.e. those that don't involve counting the frequency of a behaviour. Counting is all well and good and does serve a purpose. – just not the purported purpose. When we count stutterings in a diagnostic we assume that those counted are representative of the behaviour. The Stuttering Severity Instrument by Riley even tries to control for initial nervousness by excluding the first and last 25 words from the percentage computation. That is a well thought-out procedure. The problem here was best presented and discussed by Perkins (1990). He suggested – and was forcefully attacked by many for this – that only the person stuttering knew when stuttering was occurring; that the inherent nature of stuttering involved the involuntary aspect of the disorder. At the moment of the stuttering the person stuttering has no volitional control over the neuromuscular occurrences resulting in the stuttering. He or she is able to eventually obtain control over the musculature and either finally blurt out the sound or ease it out, or otherwise emit the sound in some fashion; but before control is established the person is not in control of his or her speech system.

This involuntary nature is supported by the information contained in this text. One is free to stop a voluntary movement; one is not free to do so when stuttering. Stuttering is the result of subcortical activity of the amygdala, hippocampus, the basal ganglia, the periaqueductal grey of the midbrain, activities of the thalamus, and finally inputs from these structures' activations into cortical areas responsible for the actual initiations of the speech and related musculature. It may therefore easily be viewed as an involuntary behaviour. So, allow the child to tell you when stuttering has occurred.

Having the child tell us results in at least three positive diagnostic pieces of information. First, it tells us immediately if or how much the child is aware of his or her dysfluencies. Second, such a procedure suggests the depth of reaction that the child is experiencing to the behaviour. If the child is reluctant to admit any difficulty or will only own up to the behaviour with prodding from the clinician, then the child is reacting in a very negative way, regardless of what few emotional reactions the child will admit to experiencing. The third positive aspect is that the procedure is undoubtedly a more accurate measure of stuttering frequency. Viewed collectively, then, the procedure results in several positives and few, if any, negatives.

What is the severity level?

The determination of severity is based on more than just the frequency count. That count can indicate the information discussed above. Severity is also a factor of the emotional reaction to speech and stuttering by the child. As such it offers a better – if more difficult to quantify – indicator of severity. Observation of the child speaking in natural settings is a good technique. Evaluation of peer reactions to the child and to his or her speech and stuttering is another. A good parent and teacher interview is a third.

Determination of struggle and secondary behaviours is also important. These indicate the extent to which the child is attempting to overcome the dysfluencies and avoid additional negative emotional reaction. The bottom line in determination of severity is an evaluation – albeit subjective – of the extent to which the child is convinced that speech is a difficult motoric behaviour to accomplish successfully. That is, how infected is the child's belief system with the virus of self-doubt and how convinced is the child that he or she is a stutterer – perhaps for now and forever? The belief system of a child is the same as the belief system of an adult. Our beliefs are determined by our experiences, by how we judge those experiences, and by how we remember those experiences. The belief system is not immutable. It can be changed if enough new positive experiences are available to lessen the impact of evaluating current behaviours through old memories. Over time the belief system calls up the more positive instead of the old negative memories and we find that our attitude about someone, something, or some activity has been altered. The same holds true for speech and stuttering. Obviously, the earlier a child who is experiencing fluency difficulties is seen in treatment the more positive the prognosis for his or her belief system concerning speech and stuttering. Altering the belief system alters the conditioned responses of the limbic and basal ganglion structures. After all, part of that conditioning involves the emotional reaction to the activity. Alter that emotional reaction and you begin to alter the conditioned behavioural responses called up by those same structures responsible for the emotional reaction. It is very cyclical; this is also why it is so important to address the belief system of the child and adult.

Unfortunately, I do not know of an instrument that singles out the evaluation of the belief system per se. That is, I don't know of an instrument that can evaluate this system at the start of a therapy process. One can infer information about the belief system from an evaluation such as is done to determine Locus of Control of Behaviour (Craig, Franklin, and Andrews, 1984). One can also conduct ongoing measures using the Self-Help Form from Ellis's Rational-Emotive Therapy technique (1977, 1984, 1986). Both of these are detailed in the following chapter on treatment. They are mentioned here because of their value in the process of ongoing diagnostics and because they can help us determine both the extent of negative beliefs and how much we have managed to change those beliefs through treatment.

Chapter Five
Treatment

Treatment for the child who stutters can incorporate any of the traditional programmes used for children. The primary difference based on this text is that treatment must not only target the behaviour of stuttering. The behaviour is just the most overt part of the problem. Underlying and maintaining this behaviour are the conditioned responses initiated by areas that also generate the emotional component of the disorder as well as contributing to the child's belief system concerning him/herself, speech, and stuttering. Any treatment must therefore also target the emotional reactions evaluated in the diagnostic, and the beliefs of the child that help reinforce conditioned responses that result in stuttering.

One of the earliest areas to be addressed should be the child's courage. Successful treatment for stuttering requires that the client be brave, that the child be able to pick himself or herself up after failure at using fluency techniques and resolve to try again after practising more. As therapists we must remember that the activities that we are requiring the child to complete are those that the child fears the most. We are asking the child to turn and face the tiger, stare him down, and make him cower – no small feats, these, especially as those are what the tiger of stuttering has always done to the child. It takes enormous courage to overcome stuttering. It takes enormous perseverance to overcome the effects of stuttering. We need to remember this every time we see our clients who stutter – children or adults.

In his treatment program, Freedom of Fluency, Daly (1988) offers some intriguing techniques applicable to both children and adults. Although he did not base the rationale for these treatments on any of the data reported in this text, the techniques do target many of the issues discussed so far. One of these techniques is motor imagery. This is not the same thing as the old progressive relaxation technique. This is the act of seeing oneself performing a behaviour perfectly in the mind's eye, the idea being that 'mental practice' could help when the behaviour is actually performed physically. Now, coaches of many different sports have used this procedure for many years mostly based on the rationale that it just 'sort of makes sense' – and it does. Very specific cortical activity is taking place when we imagine ourselves engaging in any physical activity. The areas of activity are going to sound very familiar to you since these are the supplementary motor areas, the prefrontal motor areas and subcortical areas of the basal ganglia and limbic system. In short, just about all areas involved in initiation and follow-through of any voluntary movement – with the notable exception of the primary motor strips on the frontal lobes; remember, we are imagining not performing, so the primary motor strips are not activated.

Two recent studies help shed considerable light on what is happening neurophysiologically when a client performs fluency practice through the technique of mental imagery. Decety (1996) defines motor imagery as a 'dynamic state during which representations of a given motor act are internally rehearsed in working memory without any overt motor output' (p. 45). In this review article, Decety presents evidence from several sources indicating repeated evidence that such a technique is a valuable method to increase motor learning. Skilled movements are not the only benefit of this technique. Decety reports studies that offer objective, quantified evidence that motor imaging results in significant strengthening of the involved muscles. (This may be just the evidence you need for selling that Nordic Track.)

The brain areas activated during such practice have been investigated using a variety of neuroimaging techniques including PET, MRI, rCBF, and functional MRI (fMRI) scans.

Depending on the behaviour imagined, a variety of brain areas and structures were activated during the imagery activity. These included the supplementary motor areas(s), cerebellum, anterior cingulate gyrus, prefrontal motor areas, and areas of the basal ganglia. Unfortunately, none of the behaviours included speech. One can, however, hypothesize that imagining oneself talking would also activate those areas responsible for speech. This is a reasonable conclusion since many of the areas and structures shown to activate in Decety's review also activate to support speaking.

It becomes easier to imagine how such a technique could have positive effects on a behaviour such as stuttering. Here is a technique that allows the client – child or adult – the opportunity to practise silently either fluency techniques to be used or actual fluent speech with no fear of failure. Through such practice those neural substrates of speech such as the supplementary motor areas have the opportunity to learn to respond more appropriately – i.e. with more appropriate control over the fine motor act of speaking due to no fluency-confounding subcortical input from the basal ganglia and limbic system. Smooth normal fluency may be practised that actually helps fine tune the activation of areas involved in the imagery so that, when called upon to activate in reality, they have had many hours of silent practice time.

Motor performance skill increase is great if you are a footballer but what about the autonomic responses associated with speech if you are a stutterer? For those who stutter, speaking is associated with fear and fear is associated with internal reactions such as increased respiratory rate, adrenal hormone release, cardiovascular changes and other reactions not associated with pleasure. Evaluations of autonomic responses during motor imagery tasks indicate that there is an increase in autonomic activities proportional to the imagined motor activity. There is, of course, not the same increase seen in actual motor activity but the increases are significant. For instance, Decety reported that respiration, cardiovascular rate, and systolic blood pressure all increased during imagined exercises. Respiration actually increased more during the imagined than during the actual activity. For the client who stutters, imagining speaking fluently will also result in increasingly normal autonomic responses before and during speech. Such practice could conceivably at least aid in the deconditioning of the fear response mediated by limbic-basal ganglia-cerebellar areas. The evidence definitely makes this technique one worth thinking about. Daly was wise to include it as one of many techniques in his therapy programme.

A related technique called guided visualization is used by Carl Scott (1998). His procedures are applicable to both children and adults. In guided imagery, the therapist takes a very active role by describing the scene in which the client is to visualize him or herself. This allows the practice of more appropriate emotional reactions to speaking as well as fluency practice through motor imagery. Hierarchies of stress can be determined and incorporated into the technique.

A second report by Shin et al. (1997) offers data that are very germane to the above discussion of the autonomic responses elicited by motor imagery. These authors used PET to measure rCBF in seven combat veterans with post traumatic stress disorder (PTSD) related to their experiences in Vietnam and seven controls with combat experience but no evidence of post traumatic stress disorder. During PET scans to evaluate rCBF the subjects viewed and generated visual mental images of combat.

The authors were particularly interested in rCBF in the anterior cingulate gyrus, amygdala, hippocampus and the paralimbic orbitofrontal areas. As will be discussed, the authors were surprised to find differences in rCBF in Broca's area as well in response to the visual imagery in the PTSD subjects. Results indicated that during visual imagery tasks the PTSD subjects demonstrated increased rCBF levels in the anterior cingulate gyrus, an area closely related to the limbic system and also involved in preparatory motor behaviour, especially for speech. These results occurred during imagery conditions but not during visual perception of the pictures prior to the imaging task. The focal point of rCBF was located in the ventral anterior cingulate gyrus. This is an area considered to contribute both to internal emotional states and to autonomic responses to those emotional states.

During visual imagery the PTSD group evidenced increased rCBF in the amygdala on the right. The authors remind us that the amygdala is concerned with fear conditioning and the processing of emotionally significant stimuli. Interestingly, there were no significant differences between the control group and the PTSD subjects in terms of rCBF in the orbitofrontal paralimbic regions, but remember that both had been in combat . . .

The authors were very surprised to find decreases in rCBF in Broca's area in the PTSD subjects. In the control group there were increases in rCBF to Broca's area. This decrease in Broca's area rCBF in PTSD subjects replicated the same findings in an earlier study by Rauch, Van der Kolk, Fisler, Alpert, Orr, Savage, Fischman, Jenike and Pittman (cited in Shin, 1997). The authors speculated that this decrease was the result of diminished linguistic processing whereas the PTSD subjects viewed, evaluated, and visually imagined the combat-related stimuli.

For our purposes here, the above data reinforce the idea that areas responsible for both the motoric and the emotional response are activated during imagery activities. This has some interesting treatment implications. First, by having clients who stutter imagine themselves speaking fluently in a hierarchy of stressful situations one can have them practise fluency techniques while experiencing the same general type of autonomic arousals they would actually experience. Such activities could help to lessen, or in some younger clients hopefully help extinguish, the conditioned responses related to such activities. One is pairing fluency with activities associated with dysfluency; thus we may be serving to weaken those conditioned autonomic responses associated with the fear of speaking. At the same time the client is honing the motoric skills responsible for fluent speech. It is an elegant and simple combination. It would, of course, be incorporated as a secondary procedure to the primary overt fluency training procedures of the treatment programme chosen.

It is important to understand that motor imagery differs significantly from progressive relaxation techniques. In progressive relaxation the client is talked through a series of stressful images in order to train the client to remain calm and relaxed in the face of increasingly stressful situations. As soon as the client reports any tension the relaxation procedures are instituted again. On the other hand, in motor imagery the client is internally practising the behaviour targeted, in this case fluency. The hierarchy of stressful situations is not incorporated to train relaxation but to allow the client to practise fluency in those stressful situations and despite the autonomic arousals that will result from the motor and mental imagery. Again, it could be argued that such activities could help reduce the potency of conditioned responses associated with speaking and the fear of both speech and stuttering. Such activities could be structured for use with both children and adults.

Rational emotive behaviour therapy (REBT) (Ellis, in Corsini 1984) offers some important contributions to the treatment for stuttering in both children and adults. It is a therapy based on what Ellis terms the A-B-C paradigm. An event occurs (A); an emotional response is generated (C). One assumes that the emotional response is in response to the event but Ellis reminds us that our response is also shaped by (B), our self-talk concerning the event. Our emotional reaction is the result not just of the event but also of how we talk to ourselves about what happened.

This has some serious implications in stuttering treatment, especially for generalization and maintenance. As suggested earlier, treatment should not just target the overt behaviours of stuttering but should also address the emotional reactions associated with the problem. Included in the area of emotional reactions is the belief system of the child or adult client. What we believe about our world and ourselves is partly based on what we have learned, what we have experienced, and our emotional reactions to what we have experienced. If a child or adult believes that, for him or her, talking is a difficult thing to do, that belief will be selectively matched to past experiences and will be called up when evaluating the present. If the present situation is one in which we believe we will stutter, then the chances of a stuttering moment occurring are greatly increased. If the situation does not call up that belief then the chances decrease. Some individuals who stutter in many other situations do not when they are working as disc jockeys, policemen and women, ministers or actors. They are fluent – or at least much more fluent – because their belief system does not match previous stuttering and fear of speaking with that situation or role.

Beliefs also influence success of clients at generalization and maintenance of fluency. During generalization activities the therapist requires clients to speak in situations that they have tried to actively avoid for as long as they have believed that it was a situation in which they would stutter. Suddenly, we are asking them to raise their hands in class or call the department store for information or order bacon at breakfast. They are afraid to perform these activities because they are afraid that they will stutter, that they will fail at the activity and, they tell themselves, 'That would be terrible . . .' This is where REBT can be so helpful. The techniques of REBT actively attack the inappropriate beliefs of the client. REBT refers to such beliefs as irrational and the therapist helps the client identify these irrational beliefs and replace them with rational ones. REBT maintains that irrational beliefs such as 'That would be terrible' can only lead to irrational behaviours, 'That would be terrible . . . so I can never do that . . .'; or, 'If I do raise my hand and I stutter, everyone will laugh. That would be terrible . . . I'll never be able to do this. I quit!' By identifying those beliefs as irrational and replacing those with rational beliefs, rational or desirable behaviours are more possible. An example might be the clinician responding with 'That is irrational. You might stutter, that's true. But that would not be "terrible". You've stuttered before and survived. People have laughed before and you have survived. You're here to try and I am here to help you if you fail. Failure is not the worst thing. It shows that you're trying. Refusal is worse. It tells yourself and me that you're giving up, that you're still running from the tiger . . . A more rational reaction is "I might stutter and I wouldn't like that. I would feel bad for a time and then get on with it. It tells me that I need more practice but it also tells me that I am brave enough to face my tiger. Next time I will do better."

Techniques from REBT are able to change, openly and actively, the belief system of the client by targeting the reinforcing irrational self-talk that he or she may engage in when contemplating their speech and their stutter. These techniques are not mystifying or difficult to learn and use. The chapter by Ellis in the Corsini (1984) text includes an example of the REBT Self Help Form (p.229). An example of this form as it could be used in evaluation of a generalization activity is presented below. The form is divided into A, the Activating Experience; B, Beliefs about the experience followed by rational beliefs then irrational beliefs; next is C, Consequences about your beliefs. This section is separated into desirable emotional consequences, that is, appropriate bad feelings; desirable behavioural consequences; then with inappropriate feelings and inappro- priate behaviours based on the irrational beliefs and irrational emotional reactions.

A very empowering section is the D section in which the client disputes his or her own irrational beliefs by phrasing each in the form of a question: 'Why would it be so terrible if I stuttered?'. The question form allows the client to actively dispute the specified belief. Last there are two sections in which the client lists the cognitive effects of their dispute and then the results of more appropriate feelings concerning the incident and the effect on their behaviour ('I will practise more and try again. This time I hope to do better.').

In a perfect example of how important information in one field may be overlooked by another related field, Maultsby (in Ellis and Grieger, 1977) discusses how emotional imagery can be used in REBT to heighten the experience of the procedure as well as adding realism to the cognitive evaluation of irrational versus rational reactions and responses. In this technique the client is asked to visualize the more rational behaviour and then to imagine the accompanying rational emotional reaction.

This technique was further expanded by Nardi (in Ellis and Grieger, 1986) in his chapter on the uses of psychodrama in REBT and by Dryden (in Ellis and Grieger, 1986) in her chapter, 'vivid methods in rational- emotive therapy'. Nardi borrows several techniques from Gestalt therapy in order to introduce realism into the REBT session. One of these techniques is the use of the 'double' in which either the therapist or another group member stands behind the client and voices irrational beliefs in response to rational statements being produced by the client.

RATIONAL SELF HELP FORM

Institute for Rational-Emotive Therapy   45 East 65th Street, New York 10021

INSTRUCTIONS: Please fill out the ueC section (undesirable emotional Consequences) and the ubC section (undesirable behavioral Consequences) first.
Then fill out all the A-B-C-D-E's. PLEASE PRINT LEGIBLY. BE BRIEF!

(A) ACTIVATING EXPERIENCES (OR EVENTS)

(B) BELIEFS ABOUT YOUR ACTIVATING EXPERIENCES

(C) CONSEQUENCES OF YOUR BELIEFS ABOUT ACTIVATING EXPERIENCES

(A) ACTIVATING EXPERIENCES:
TRANSFER ACTIVITY. COULDN'T USE EASY ONSET WHEN VOLUNTEERING AN ANSWER IN CLASS AND I STUTTERED. SOME KIDS LAUGHED AT ME

(rB) rational Beliefs (your wants or desires)
I WISH I HAD DONE BETTER. I DON'T LIKE BEING LAUGHED AT. THIS MAY BE HARDER THAN I THOUGHT.

(iB) Irrational Beliefs (your demands or commands)
I'LL NEVER BE ABLE TO USE EASY ONSET. IT WAS TERRIBLE WHEN EVERYONE LAUGHED. I'M SO STUPID. I'LL NEVER TALK RIGHT.

(deC) desirable emotional Consequences (appropriate bad feelings)
I WAS DISAPPOINTED. I WAS SAD.

(dbC) desirable behavioral Consequences (desirable behaviors)
I NEED TO WORK HARDER—MORE PRACTICE. NEXT TIME I'LL SHOW THEM I CAN

(ueC) undesirable emotional Consequences (inappropriate feelings)
I WAS DEPRESSED FOR DAYS. I FELT STUPID & WORTHLESS

(ubC) undesirable behavioral Consequences (undesirable behaviors)
I'LL NEVER RAISE MY HAND AGAIN. I'LL NEVER DO ANOTHER ACTIVITY.

(D) DISPUTING OR DEBATING YOUR IRRATIONAL BELIEFS
(State this in the form of questions)
IS IT TOO HARD TO EVER DO AGAIN? WHY WOULDN'T I EVER BE ABLE TO USE EASY ONSET? WAS IT SO TERRIBLE WHEN "EVERYONE" LAUGHED? AM I SO STUPID? WILL I NEVER TALK RIGHT?

(E) EFFECTS OF DISPUTING OR DERATING YOUR IRRATIONAL BELIEFS

(cE) cognitive Effects of disputing (similar to rational beliefs)
THE FIRST TIME WAS DIFFICULT BUT EASY ONSET IS NOT TOO HARD TO EVER DO AGAIN. I CAN USE EASY ONSET AND WITH MORE PRACTICE I WILL BE ABLE TO USE IT WHEN I NEED TO. I WILL NEVER LIKE IT WHEN PEOPLE LAUGH BUT I CAN TAKE IT. I'M NOT STUPID. I'M TRYING TO DO ANOTHER ACTIVITY. I WILL TALK BETTER IF I PRACTICE AND AM COURAGEOUS

(eE) emotional Effects (appropriate feelings)
I FELT SAD BUT I WON'T BE DEPRESSED. I WAS DISAPPOINTED BUT I'M NOT SO OK. I'M NOT WORTHLESS

(bE) behavioral Effects (desirable behaviors)
I RAISED MY HAND AGAIN AND DID BETTER BECAUSE I PRACTICED MORE. I AM PRACTICING MY NEXT "TRANSFER ACTIVITY" AND FEEL MORE CONFIDENT, EVEN IF THE NEXT TIME'S NOT BEST

Figure 5.1: REBT self-help form.

The client then responds with immediate rational answers. Another such technique is the 'empty chair', long a staple in the therapeutic armoury of Gestalt therapy. Here the client engages himself or herself in a debate about the results of some behavioural change. As the client adopts each persona he or she changes chairs and argues back at the 'empty chair' that just previously contained the alternative persona. One can imagine the kind of dialogue that a client who stutters might have with his or her alternative personas of 'I, the stutter' and 'I, who am in therapy to become fluent':

> I, the stutter: ' How dare you! How could you get rid of me? I have kept you safe for years. I kept you from trying those ridiculous plans of yours that could have failed and hurt you. How could you be so stupid? I've been a part of you longer than you can remember . . .'

> I, who am in therapy to become fluent: 'You never kept me safe! I'm not stupid! What I am is sick of you! I'm going to do everything I can to get you out of my life!'

Dryden describes a technique that is probably more accessible to speech therapists. She suggests that the client write a scenario describing not just the situation but including the imagined dialogue that client could have with individuals in the scene ('Oh no – he isn't going to subject me to that again, is he?') In this exercise the client is told to be as realistic and brutal as possible, to compose the worst case scenario and have the participants say the worst things that can be imagined to him or her. A therapist can assume that an individual who stutters – especially an older child or adult – would have, unfortunately, little difficulty generating such an assignment. In the REBT session the therapist can give voice to the other parts. The client then evaluates irrational emotional and behavioural reactions and replaces these with rational counterparts.

REBT may seem to be most applicable to older children and adults but that is really not the case. There are specific adaptations of the techniques for younger children as well. Play therapy procedures can be incorporated. 'Toughening' exercises can be practised in the safety of the clinical environment and emotional reactions that only serve to strengthen conditioned emotional and behavioural reactions can be attacked and hopefully weakened.

Once a generalization technique has been practised enough and the client is ready to make the attempt to incorporate it outside the safe world of the clinic, the use of behavioural contracts can be of benefit. Behavioural contracting is nothing new. These have been a core technique of reality therapy for years as well as an important component of more recent therapies for stuttering such as presented by Daly and earlier by Shames and Florence (1980). These contracts spell out exactly what the client expects of himself or herself – not what the clinician expects. This is an important differentiation. The behaviour to be completed must be the responsibility of the client. Before setting out REBT can be very useful in identifying beliefs that will be counterproductive. Rational emotive behaviour therapy visualization and psychodramas can be generated to prepare the client for rational and productive pre- and post-reactions. 'Failure' can be discussed as well as success. We want to change both behaviour and emotion in order to effect a neurological change. Both emotion and behaviour affect beliefs and it is the belief system of the client that is contributing so heavily to reinforcement of the inappropriate neurological component that forms the basis of stuttering. Therefore, inappropriate beliefs in the adult client must be identified and changed. A child's belief system beginning to become infected with inappropriate beliefs concerning themselves or attitudes about speaking must also be targeted. Such belief systems become self-reinforcing and serve to reinforce the conditioned fear responses and inappropriate reactions of subcortical and cortical speech initiation and control centres. Rational emotive behaviour therapy and behavioural contracting can both be of real help and of real service to our clients who stutter, whether children or adults.

In his excellent text, *Clinical Decision Making in the Diagnosis and Treatment of Fluency Disorders* (1996), Manning presents an interesting summary of the Locus of Control of Behaviour (Craig et al. 1984). The LCB, as it is called, is a 17-item Likert-type inventory. The purpose of the LCB is to help determine how able a person is to maintain a newly acquired or desired behaviour. A high score indicates that the client is more externally controlled, a lower score indicates the opposite – that the client is maintaining responsibility for his or her new skill and maintenance of it. Generalization and maintenance of a new skill such as fluency is best accomplished and maintained if an individual is internally responsible for that activity. The individual is less at the mercy of the environment because he or she is monitoring and reinforcing the new behaviour. The LCB is an appealing instrument to include in diagnostics and as a partial indicator of both treatment efficacy and as a prognostic indicator for success in generalization activities as well as success at longer term maintenance. The abilities of the LCB to tell us these things are reportedly mixed (Manning, 1996); however, the LCB is recommended here because of its ease of administration, scoring and interpretation. It is also recommended due to its inferential capabilities. A client whose behaviour is externally controlled has not addressed his or her belief system sufficiently.

Recall the discussion of REBT above. Irrational thoughts often involve the anticipation or interpretation of the reactions of others to their speech ('everyone would laugh and that would be terrible'). This would suggest that individuals have not sufficiently internalized their locus of control. It is anticipated that clients who demonstrate rational beliefs concerning themselves, stuttering, speech, generalization and maintenance activities, would score low on the LCB, indicating a more internally controlled acquisition and maintenance of behaviour. Such a score might also indicate a potential for lessened conditioned negative response to speaking.

In summary, the information from this text suggests the following concerning diagnosis and treatment of stuttering in both children and adults:

1. Diagnostics should consist of considerably more than frequency counts. Allow the client to indicate a stuttering moment.
2. Evaluate the emotional reaction of the client to both speech and to stuttering.
3. Administer the Locus of Control of Behaviour test (Craig et al., 1984) as one of the baseline measurements for effectiveness of treatment of the belief system.
4. Administer the Self Help Form of the REBT technique (Ellis, in Corsini, 1984) as an ongoing diagnostic and treatment instrument for evaluation of belief system and change.
5. Incorporate motor imaging exercises with emotional concurrence as a standard treatment protocol.

Last, allow me the opportunity to state the obvious. An effective therapist is not a friend. Therapists can and should be empathetic, warm, concerned and all those other adjectives that are so soft and fuzzy, but not a friend. An effective therapist is a motivator, a confronter and, yes, a task driver. Few clients in physical therapy consider their therapists as friends. After a knee surgery that required weeks of physical therapy my brother, only half joking, stills refers to his physical therapist as his 'physical terrorist' – but he walks better and with far less pain. Now before you start to write letters, let me say that I am not proposing that we change our moniker or conduct therapy as speech-language terrorists. What I am saying is that our clients who stutter – *especially* our clients who stutter – do not need the sympathy of a friend. Better their fluency improve and they never send us Christmas cards than they become more 'comfortable' with their stutter and never be fluent.

Afterword

The preceding information and inference present some interesting questions for future research. Some of these questions might include the following:

1. Some data from studies examining the autonomic responses of subjects who stutter report no such unusual arousals in adult subjects who stutter, either before or during the stuttering event (Miller, 1993). The procedures used to evaluate these responses were not invasive and could be easily adapted to children. Based on the preceding information, it would be interesting to investigate whether children exhibit the same lack of significant autonomic arousals before and during stuttering. It would be predicted that autonomic arousal in children who stutter would be significantly higher than the responses obtained in some adults as the children are in the process of acquiring conditioned fear responses to the act of speaking whereas the adults have lived and coped with those same conditioned responses over a number of years. One could infer from the results whether a kindling type of phenomenon was occurring in the non-emotional stuttering of adults in previous studies. One might also be able to detect the autonomic activities associated with the acquisition of a fear-related conditioned response to the act of speaking in the children. Prevention and treatment measures might be able to be generated based on such results.

2. Dopamine uptake has been associated with several of the studies presented and reviewed in this book. Haloperidol, a dopamine-uptake blocker, has been reported by some to act to reduce the frequency and severity of stuttering. Increased dopamine levels have also been found to be associated with stuttering. Parkinson's disease is a problem of insufficient dopamine availability for use by the basal ganglia. It would be intriguing to survey a sample of Parkinson patients to determine if those among them who stuttered found that the frequency and severity of the stutter declined as the disease progressed. Conversely, did the dopamine replacement therapy have any effect on their stutter? Did the

stutter return to pre-Parkinson's levels? Did stuttering that had lessened with age re-emerge as a result of increased dopamine availability and uptake?

3. Motor imagery is associated with increases in both skill level of those activities imagined and with increased mass of muscles involved in completion of that imagined activity. It might be valuable to investigate this type of skill practice as a therapy technique for stuttering, especially after a PET scan study, to see what structures and areas are activated during imagined fluency and during remembered episodes of stuttering.

4. During the investigation of number three above it would be interesting to record any instances of autonomic arousal associated with imagined stuttering. If the motor imagery results in all aspects of the behaviour, including increased heart rate, respiratory rate and the like, then other physiological changes associated with emotional arousal should be available for recording as well.

5. A well-controlled study of treatment efficacy of motor imagery.

6. PET scans of controls and subjects who stutter. These scans could be done under four conditions: while the subjects who stutter are silent and at rest; just prior to the speech attempt; during the actual stuttering event; and during silence following the stuttering event. Such scans would allow investigation of structures and areas suggested in this text as contributing to the stuttering, especially those activated during speech onset.

7. Researchers in stuttering need to become more familiar with the concept of long-term potentiation (LTP) as it relates to conditioned responses. The kindling phenomenon is a basic starting point as both it and LTP appear to result in the same types of response. The fact that research shows that a small amount of stimulation can result in as great a response as a large amount of stimulation has serious implications for the explanation of stuttering. If it can be demonstrated that conditioned fear responses mediated by the amygdala, a structure very susceptible to both kindling and long-term potentiation, can result from minimal stimuli once those reactions are learned, a possible road to experimentally explaining so-called non-emotional stuttering could begin. With apologies to my behaviouristic friends, behaviour is the end product and we need to focus on the cellular processes causing the behaviour.

8. Studies replicating those of Wu and his colleagues, who reported high dopamine and low activations of cortical/subcortical limbic and motor areas in SWS.

The above is, of course, not a complete list of the questions raised by the information in this text but just reflects general areas for possible future research.

One concern experienced while researching this book was the enormous amount of information out there. Most of the data that are germane to the neurology of stuttering are found in journals other than those typically associated with speech pathology. The task of the next researcher is to evaluate and correlate neurological research published both inside and also, and particularly, outside the field of speech pathology beginning in 1998.

Appendix
Connections of the amygdala

Subcortical connections

Striatum (Halgren, 1995: p. 30)

- 'Substantial' amygdaloid projection to ventral parts of striatum (especially nucleus accumbens and olfactory tubercle).
- The amygdala also projects to dorsal and caudal parts of striatum.
- Some amygdaloid projections terminate in the ventral and medial parts of the caudate nucleus and putamen that border the nucleus accumbens.
- However, many amygdalostriatal fibres extend to the caudal part of the ventral putamen, dorsal to the amygdala, and to the entire extent of the body and tail of the caudate nucleus, bordering the stria terminalis (considered one of the most substantial efferents of the amygdala). It originates predominately from the basal and accessory basal nuclei.
- Amygdala projects to the ventral pallidum (this projection is 'light' compared to striatal areas).
- Direct projection from amygdala to mediodorsal nucleus.
- Nucleus accumbens (which has strong amygdala input) has a substantial projection to the ventral pallidum.

Basal forebrain (Halgren, 1995: p.31)

- Amygdaloid projection is directed heavily (but not only) to the major components of the magnocellular basal forebrain nuclei (MBFN).
- Very few cells that project to the cholinergic basal forebrain are located in the magnocellular division of the basal nucleus, which receives the largest input from the basal forebrain. These fibres do not terminate in the forebrain.
- The projection from the MBFN to the amygdala arises mainly from the anterolateral part of the nucleus basalis.

Diencephalon

Thalamus (Halgren, 1992; p. 33)

- The central and medial nuclei of the amygdala project to the midline thalamic nuclei (superior, inferior, and densocellular of the nucleus centralis of Olszewski).
- Afferent to amygdala from thalamus – mediodorsal nucleus of thalamus does not reciprocate the connection to the amygdala.
- Thalamoamygdaloid connections arise from the midline thalamic nuclei (the same ones that receive connections from the amygdala).
- The parvicellular part of the ventroposterior nucleus of the thalamus also projects to the amygdala (in rats and cats).
- The posterior part of thalamus in/around medial geniculate nucleus has substantial inputs to the thalamus (in rats and cats).
- 'These posterior thalamic areas receive auditory inputs from the inferior colliculus and the pathway to the amygdala has been implicated in conditioned emotional responses to auditory stimuli'.

Hypothalamus

- The bed nucleus provides a relay for projections from the amygdala to the hypothalamus and brain stem (as do the central and medial nuclei).
- Some fibres going from the amygdala to the bed nucleus travel through the stria terminalis; others go through the amygdalofugal pathway.
- The central and basal nuclei of the amygdala project to the lateral part of the bed nucleus.
- The medial and posterior cortical nuclei of the amygdala and the amygdalohippocampal area project to the medial bed nucleus.
- Fibres originating in the anterior cortical and medial nuclei appear to terminate in the anterior hypothalamus.
- A substantial amygdaloid projection terminates in and around the ventromedial hypothalamic nucleus (divided into two components) and the premammillary nuclei.
- The amygdala projects to the full rostrocaudal extent of the lateral hypothalamus. The connection begins mainly in the central nucleus (with minor contributions from medial and anterior cortical nuclei) and most fibres travel to the hypothalamus through the ventral amygdalofugal pathway. Some fibres travel in the stria terminalis.
- Afferent connections to amygdala from hypothalamus – most arise in the ventromedial hypothalamic nucleus and other caudal areas of lateral hypothalamic areas and travel to central, medial, and accessory basal nuclei and parvicellular division of the basal nucleus.

Brain stem (Halgren, 1992: p. 35)

- Central nucleus of the amygdala sends fibres into and through midbrain, pons, and medulla, and spinal cord.
- No other amygdaloid nuclei contribute to this projection (but bed nucleus of stria terminalis has a similar projection).
- '. . . the fibres innervate a number of structures that have been implicated in autonomic control, including periaqueductal grey, parabrachial nucleus, dorsal vagal nuclei, and reticular formation.' (p. 35).
- In the midbrain, the central nucleus projects to the ventral tegmental area and substantia nigra (lateral part of the pars compacta).
- The central nucleus extends into the peripeduncular nucleus and tegmental reticular formation, then dorsomedially into periaqueductal grey.
- The central nucleus projection continues through pontine reticular formation, and terminates heavily in the parabrachial nuclei located around superior cerebellar peduncle. Some fibres extend medially into the nucleus raphe magnus.
- In the medulla, the central nucleus projection is dispersed to the lateral part of the reticular formation (most heavily into the nucleus of the solitary tract and the dorsal motor nucleus of the vagus).
- Afferent to amygdala from brain stem – the amygdaloid projection to dorsal pons is reciprocated by fibres from the parabrachial nucleus which end in the central nucleus.
- Noradrenergic input terminates in the central and basal amygdaloid nuclei.
- The nucleus of the solitary tract (in primates) projects to the parabrachial nuclei, which (as stated above) projects to the amygdala.
- Connections with the olfactory system (pp. 35–6).

Hippocampus/hippocampal formation

- Primary interaction between the hippocampal formation and the amygdala is through the entorhinal cortex. From the amygdaloid complex, the entorhinal cortex receives projections from the lateral nucleus, accessory basal nucleus, periamygdaloid cortex, anterior cortical and medial nuclei, and the paralaminar nucleus.
- Only rostral portion of the entorhinal cortex receives a major amygdaloid projection.
- Largest input to entorhinal cortex is from the lateral nucleus.
- Next largest input to entorhinal cortex is from the accessory basal nucleus.
- Dentate gyrus does not appear to receive input from the amygdala.
- An amygdaloid projection beginning in the magnocellular division of

the accessory basal nucleus travels ventrally to the hippocampal formation.

- Another amygdaloid projection, beginning mainly from the parvicellular division of the basal nucleus and from the periamygdaloid cortex, terminates at the border of field CA1 and the subiculum.
- Afferent to amygdala from hippocampal formation, fibres from the entorhinal cortex pass through the lateral cortex in route to the substantia innominata and other basal forebrain regions; this provides the potential to communicate with cells in the nucleus. However, these fibres' characteristics (coarse and smooth) do not contribute to diffuse terminal plexus in the lateral nucleus.
- The rostrocaudal extent of hippocampus provides some cells that give rise to projections to the amygdala. These are located along the border of the subiculum and CA1. These few cells connect to the parvicellular division of the basal nucleus and to the periamygdaloid cortex.

Cortical connections of the amygdala

Temporal and occipital lobe connections

Visual connections

- The anterior part of the inferotemporal cortex (TE) connects with the amygdala and appears to be the major route of entry for unimodal visual information to the amygdala.
- It is unclear whether or not all portions of the TE project to the amygdala.
- It appears that most of the inferior temporal cortex (located anterior to the rostral limit of the occipital temporal sulcus) does contribute to the amygdaloid projection.
- Projections from the caudal levels of the TE terminate exclusively in the dorsal half of the lateral nucleus of the amygdala.
- Projections from more rostral levels of TE (especially ventromedial portion) terminate in the dorsal tip of the magnocellular division of the basal nucleus.

Auditory connections

- Not as well defined as visual connections.
- Turner and co-workers, cited in Halgren (1992) found no degeneration of the amygdala following selective lesions of primary auditory and surrounding cortex. These lesions did lead to projections to more rostral levels of the superior temporal gyrus (which projects to the ventrolateral portion of the lateral nucleus).
- There is little physiological evidence, but some anatomical evidence

exists supporting the idea that the rostral portion of the superior temporal gyrus may function as a unimodal auditory association cortex. Therefore, projections from this area may provide major auditory input to the amygdala.

Polysensory connections

- Medial and lateral portions of the temporal pole contribute projections to the amygdala.
- The projection is heaviest to the lateral nucleus and focused in the ventromedial portion of the nucleus.
- The accessory basal nucleus (especially magnocellular division) receives prominent projection.
- The parvicellular division of the basal nucleus has a more modest connection.
- More caudal areas of the perirhinal cortex (areas 36r and 36c) project to the amygdala in a decreased projection that is distributed exclusively to the lateral nucleus.
- The amygdala connects to almost all levels of the visual cortex (in the monkey).
- Based on fluorescent tracer injection studies, the amygdala appears to connect to all portions of visually related temporal and occipital neocortex.
- The projection is distributed in gradient fashion (the heaviest projections going to anterior temporal lobe and progressively lighter toward more caudal levels of the visual cortex).
- Projections to caudal levels originate exclusively from the basal nucleus (especially magnocellular division).
- Projections to rostral levels of the inferior temporal cortex also originate in the accessory basal ganglia.
- Using two tracers in experiments has shown that largely independent populations of cells in the basal ganglia project to different parts of the visual cortex.
- The cells in the basal nucleus that project to the visual cortex receive either no direct visual input (intermediate and parvicellular divisions) or very little input from the most rostral levels of the temporal lobe (magnocellular division).
- The amygdala projects to the rostral half of the superior temporal gyrus; these projections extend back (very lightly) into primary auditory cortex and immediately adjacent association cortex.
- A much heavier projection is directed to more rostral levels of the superior temporal gyrus than to the caudal periauditory regions.
- The amygdala projects heavily to the temporal polar cortex. The projection is heavier to the medial, perirhinal portion of the temporal pole than the projection to the lateral component. These projections origi-

nate mainly from the lateral and accessory basal nuclei (few or none originate in the basal nucleus).

Frontal, insular, and cingulate connections

- Agranular insula extends rostrally to occupy the caudal part of the orbital cortex (subdivided into Iav, Iad, Iap, and Ias). All of these areas are densely innervated by the amygdala (but different amygdaloid nuclei).
- Lateral orbital cortex (mostly area 12) and medial orbital cortex (Walker's are 14 and part of 13) along with Walker's original areas (13a and 13b) receive substantial amygdaloid projection; 13 proper receives very little amygdaloid innervation.
- Medial wall of the hemisphere (areas 24, 25, 32, and area 24 of the anterior cingulate gyrus) receive amygdaloid input.
- Projections to the insula fade out caudally through the dysgranular and granular fields.
- Projections to the orbital cortex and medial wall diminish over rostral parts of areas 12, 14, 24 and 32 and fade out laterally toward the principal sulcus.
- Projection to the cingulate gyrus decreases caudally toward area 23.
- Amygdaloid projections seems to be absent in area 10 ; areas 11 and 13 receive only light, patchy input, and dorsolateral regions of prefrontal cortex (areas 8, 9, 45, 46, premotor cortex – 6) receive only patchy, insubstantial input.

Projections to the amygdala

- The rostral insula projects heavily to the dorsomedial part of the lateral nucleus, parvicellular division of basal nucleus, and medial nucleus; the posterior insula projects almost exclusively to the lateral nucleus.
- Caudal insular projection may provide a major route for somatosensory information to reach the amygdala. The second somatosensory area is reciprocally connected with the granular and dysgranular insular cortices. (These provide the most direct route as these regions both connect with the lateral nucleus.)
- These regions of the lateral nucleus that receive input from the insula do not give rise to projections back to the insula.
- The caudal orbital cortex projects to the basal nucleus, magnocellular division of the accessory basal nucleus and the dorsomedial portion of the lateral nucleus.
- There is some evidence that the rostral insula and caudal orbital cortex may project to the central nucleus.
- The cingulate gyrus projects to the magnocellular division of the basal nucleus.
- The medial wall of the prefrontal cortex projects to both the magnocel-

lular divisions of the basal and accessory basal nuclei.
- The amygdala can also influence the frontal cortex through its connections with the thalamus. It projects to the mediodorsal thalamic nucleus, which connects with the frontal cortex.
- The projection to the mediodorsal thalamic nucleus arises from almost all of the amygdaloid nuclei but especially the lateral, basal, and accessory basal nuclei and the periamygdaloid cortex.
- Exceptions to the connections may be the central and media nuclei since most of these fibres end in the midline thalamic nucleus located medial to the mediodorsal thalamic nucleus.

References

Abe K, Yokoyama SY, Yorifuji S (1993) Repetitive speech disorder resulting from infarcts in the paramedian thalami and midbrain. Journal of Neurology, Neurosurgery and Psychiatry 56: 1024–6.

Amaral D (1993) Emotional neurophysiology of the amygdala within the context of human cognition. In JP Aggleton (ed.) The Amygdala. New York: John Wiley & Sons.

Arnold, MB (1970) Brain function in emotion: a phenomenologic analysis. In P Black (ed.) Physiologic correlates of emotion. New York: Academic Press, pp. 261–84.

Bard P (1929) The central representation of the sympathetic nervous system as indicated by certain physiologic observations. Archives of Neurological Psychiatry 22: 230–46.

Bard P (ed.) (1961) Medical physiology. St Louis: CV Mosby.

Bhatnager S, Andy O (1989) Alleviation of stuttering with human centremedian thalamic stimulation. Journal of Neurosurgery and Psychiatry 52(10): 1182–4.

Borden G, Harris K (1980) Speech Science Primer. Baltimore: Williams & Wilkins.

Botez MI, Barbeau A (1971) Role of subcortical structures, and particularity of the thalamus, in the mechanisms of speech and language. International Journal of Neurology 8: 2– 4.

Brutten EJ, Shoemaker D (1967) The modification of stuttering. Englewood Cliffs NJ: Prentice-Hall.

Brutten EJ, Shoemaker, D (1971) A two factor theory of stuttering. In LE Travis (ed.) Handbook of speech pathology and audiology. Englewood Cliffs NJ: Prentice-Hall.

Cannon WB (1927) The James – Lange theory of emotion: a critical examination and an alternative theory. American Journal of Psychology 39: 106–25.

Chimelova A (1975) In M Lastovka (1995) Tremor in stutterers. Folia Phonoiatr Logop 47: 318–23.

Ciemins VA (1970) Localized thalamic hemorrhage: a cause of aphasia. Neurology 20: 776–82.

Clark WEL (1950) Relationships between the cerebral cortex and the hypothalamus. British Medical Bulletin 6: 341.

Connor NP, Abbs JH (1990) Sensorimotor contributions of the basal ganglia: recent advances. Physical Therapy 70 (12): 118–28.

Corsini R (ed.) (1984) Current Psychotherapies. Itasca IL: FE Peacock.

Craig A, Franklin J, Andrews G (1984) A scale to measure locus of control of behavior. British Journal of Medical Psychology 57: 176–80.

Daly DA (1988) The Freedom of Fluency: A Therapy Program for the Chronic Stutterer. Moline IL: LinguiSystems Inc.

Damasio A (1984) Disturbances of personality, affect, mood, intellect and movement secondary to frontal lobe damage: Implications for autism, attention, and learning disorders. Neurological Foundations of Behavior. Symposium conducted in Oakland, California.

Darley FL, Aronson AE, Brown JR (1975) Motor Speech Disorders. Philadelphia: WB Saunders Co.

Davis M (1992) The role of the amygdala in conditioned fear. In JP Aggleton (ed.) The Amygdala. New York: John Wiley & Sons, pp. 255–306.

Decety J (1996) The neurophysiological basis of motor imagery. Behavioural Brain Research 77: 45–52.

Denny M, Smith A (1997) Respiratory and laryngeal control in stuttering. In RF Curlee, GM Seigel (eds), Nature and Treatment of Stuttering. Needham Heights, MA: Allyn & Bacon.

Egger MD (1972) Amygdaloid-hypothalamic neurophysiological interrelationships in the neurobiology of the amygdala. In BE Eleftheriou (ed.) The Neurobiology of the Amygdala. New York: Plenum Press, pp. 261–93.

Egger MD, Flynn JP (1963) Effects of electrical stimulation of the amygdala on hypothalamically elicited attack behavior in cats. Journal of Neurophysiology 26: 705–20.

Ellis A (1984) Rational-emotive therapy. In R Corsini (ed.) Current Psychotherapies. Ithaca, NY: FE Peacock, pp. 196–236.

Ellis A, Grieger R (eds) (1977) A Handbook of Rational Emotive Therapy. New York: Springer Publications.

Ellis A, Grieger R (1986) Handbook of Rational-Emotive Therapy: Volume Two. New York: Springer Publications.

Fox PT, Ingham RJ, Ingham JC, Hirsch TB, Downs JH, Martin C, Jerabek P, Glass T, Lancaster JL (1996) A PET study of the neural systems of stuttering. Nature 382: 158–62.

Fried I, Wilson C, MacDonald K, Behnke EJ (1998) Electrical current stimulates laughter. Nature 391: 650–1.

Gatz AJ (1970) Clinical neuroanatomy and neurophysiology. Philadelphia: FA Davis.

Gellhorn E, Loofborrow GN (1963) Emotions and disorders. New York: Harper & Row.

Geschwind N (1968) Human brain: left-right asymmetries in temporal speech regions. Science 161: 186–7.

Gloor P (1972) Temporal lobe epilepsy: its possible contribution to the understanding of the functional significance of the amygdala and of its interaction with neocortical-temporal mechanisms. In BE Eleftheriou (ed.) The Neurobiology of the Amygdala New York: Plenum Press, pp. 296–315.

Gloor P (1978) Inputs and outputs of the amygdala: what the amygdala is trying to tell the rest of the brain. In KE Livingston, D Hornydiewicz (eds) Limbic Mechanisms. New York: Plenum Press, pp. 189–211.

Gloor P (1997) The Temporal Lobe and Limbic System. New York: Oxford University Press.

Goldberg G (1985) Supplementary motor area structure and function: review and hypotheses. The Behavioral and Brain Sciences 8: 567–616.

Guiot G, Hertzog E, Rondot P, Molina P (1961) Arrest or acceleration of speech evoked by thalamic stimulation in the course of stereotaxic procedures for parkinsonism. Brain 84: 363–9.

Guyton AC (ed.) (1976) Textbook of medical physiology. Philadelphia: WB Saunders.

Halgren E (1992) Emotional neurophysiology of the amygdala within the context of human cognition. In JP Aggleton (ed.) The Amygdala. New York: John Wiley & Sons, pp. 191–228.

Ham R (1986) Techniques of stuttering therapy. Englewood Cliffs NJ: Prentice-Hall.

Hammond LJ (1970) Conditioned emotional states. In P Black (ed.) Physiological Correlates of Emotion. New York: Academic Press, pp. 245–58.

Hassler R (1966) Thalamus regulation of muscle tone and speed movements. In D Purpura, M Yahr (eds) The Thalamus. New York: Columbia University Press, pp. 36–51.

Ingham RJ, Fox PT, Ingham JC (1994) Brain image investigation of the speech of stutterers and nonstutterers. ASHA 36: 188.

Ingham RJ, Fox PT, Ingham JC, Zamarripa F, Martin C, Jerabek P, Cotton J (1996) Functional-lesion investigation of developmental stuttering with positron emission tomography. Journal of Speech and Hearing Research 39: 1208–27.

Isaacson RL (1974) The Limbic System. New York: Plenum Press.

James W (1884) What is emotion? Mind 9: 118–205.

Jasper HH, Rasmussen T (1958) Studies of clinical and electrical responses to deep temporal stimulation in men with some considerations of functional anatomy. Research Publications of the Association of Research in Nervous and Mental Disease 36: 316–34.

Jonas S (1982) The thalamus and aphasia, including transcortical aphasia: a review. Journal of Communication Disorders 15: 31–41.

Jones EG, Powell TPS (1970) Cortical association connections. Brian 93: 793–820.

Joseph R (1982) The neurophysiology of development: Hemispheric laterality, limbic language and the origin of thought. Journal of Clinical Psychology 38(1): 4–33.

Jurgens U (1969) The cingulate gyrus. Experimental Brain Research 9: 554–60.

Jurgens U (1994) The role of the periaqueductal grey in vocal behaviour. Behavioural Brain Research 62: 107–17.

Jurgens U, Muller-Preuss P (1977) Convergent projections of different limbic vocalization areas in the squirrel monkey. Experimental Brain Research 29: 75–83.

Jurgens U, Von Cremon D (1982) On the role of the anterior cingulate cortex in phonation: a case report. Brain and Language 15(2): 234–48.

Jurgens U, Zwirer P (1996) The role of the periaqueductal gray and neocortical vocal fold control. Neuroreport 7(18): 2921–3.

Kaada BR (1951) Somato-motor, autonomic and electro corticographic responses to electrical stimulation in primates, cats, and dogs. Acta Physiologica Scandanavia 83 (Suppl.): 1–285.

Kaada BR (1967) Brain mechanisms related to aggressive behavior. In CD Clemente and PB Lindsley (eds), Aggression and Defense. Berkeley: University Press, pp. 118–31.

Kaada BR (1972) Stimulation and regional ablation of the amygdaloid complex with reference to functional representations. In BE Eleftheriou (ed.) The Neurobiology of the Amygdala. New York: Plenum Press, pp. 211–28.

Kapp BS, Whalen PJ, Supple W, Pascoe JP (1992) Projections of the amygdala. In JP Aggleton (ed.) The Amygdala. New York: John Wiley & Sons Inc.

Kidd K (1984) Stuttering as a genetic disorder. In RF Curlee, WH Perkins (eds) Nature and Treatment of Stuttering: New Directions. Boston: Allyn & Bacon, pp. 149–69.

Kimura M (1995) Role of basal ganglia in behavioral learning. Neuroscience Research 22: 353–8.

Kirshner MS, Kistler KH (1982) Aphasia after right thalamic hemorrhage. Archives of Neurology 39(10): 667–9.

Lalonde R, Botez MI (1990) The cerbellum and learning processes in animals. Brain Res Rev 15: 325–32.

Lange CG (1969) Über Gemutsbewegungen. In MB Arnold (ed.) The Nature of Emotion. Baltimore: Penguin Books.

Larsen BS, Lassen NA (1978) Variations in regional cortical blood flow in the right and left hemispheres during automatic speech. Brain 101: 193–209.

Lastovka M (1995) Tremor in Stutterers. Folia Phoniatr Logop 47: 318–23.

LeDoux JE (1993a) Emotional memory systems in the brain. Behavioural Brain Research 58: 69–79.

LeDoux JE (1993b) Emotional memory: In search of systems and synapses. Annals New York Academy of Sciences 702: 149–57.

Leiner HC, Leiner AL, Dow RS (1991) The human cerebro-cerebellar system: its computing, cognitive, and language skills. Behavioural Brain Research 44: 113–28.

Lindsley DB (1970) The role of nonspecific reticulo-thalamocortical systems in emotion. In P Black (ed.) Physiological Correlates of Emotion. New York: Academic Press, pp. 147–84.

Livingston KE (ed.) (1976) Limbic Mechanisms. New York: Plenum Press.

MacLean PD (1954) The limbic system and its hippocampal formation: Studies in animals and their possible application to man. Journal of Neurosurgery 11: 29–44.

MacLean PD (1970) The limbic brain in relation to the psychoses. In P Black (ed.) Physiological Correlates of Emotion New York: Academic Pressm, pp. 130–44.

Manning WH (1996) Clinical decision making in the diagnosis and treatment of fluency disorders. Albany, New York: Delmar Publishers.

McKeough DM (1982) The Coloring Review of Neuroscience. Boston: Little, Brown.

Miller S (1993) Multiple measures of anxiety and psychophysiologic arousal in stutterers and nonstutterers during nonspeech and speech tasks of increasing complexity. Unpublished doctoral dissertation, University of Texas at Dallas, Richardson.

Mullan S, Penfield W (1959) Illusions of comparative interpretation and emotion. Archives of Neurological Psychiatry 81: 269–76.

Nauta WJH (1962) Neural associations of the amygdaloid complex in the monkey. Brain 85: 595.

Nolte J (1993) The Human Brain (3rd edn) St Louis, MO: Mosby Year-Book.

Ojemann GA, Fedio P, Van Buren JM (1968) Anomia from pulvinar and subcortical parietal stimulation. Brain 91: 99–116.

Ojemann GA, Ward AA (1971) Speech representation in the ventrolateral thalamus. Brain 94: 669–80.

Orton S, Travis LE (1929) Studies in stuttering: studies of action currents in stutterers. Archives of Neurological Psychiatry 21: 61–8.

Papez JW (1937) A proposed mechanism of emotion. Archives of Neurologic Psychiatry 38: 725–43.

Penfield W (1950) The supplementary motor area in the cerebral cortex of man. Archives of Psychiatry 85: 670–4.

Penfield W, Roberts L (1959) Speech and Brain Mechanisms. Princeton, NJ: Princeton University Press.

Perkins WH (1990) What is stuttering? Journal of Speech and Hearing Research 55: 370–82.

Physicians Desk Reference (1996) Oradell, NJ: Medical Economics Co.

Pool KD, Devous MD, Freeman FJ, Watson BC, Finitzo T (1991) Regional cerebral blood flow in developmental stutterers. Archives of Neurology 48: 509–12.

Roberts WW, Steinberg MC, Means LW (1976) Hypothalamic mechanisms for sexual, aggressive, and other motivational behaviors in the opossum, Dedelphis, Virginia. Journal of Comparative Physiological Psychology 64: 1–15.

Robinson, B. W (1967) Vocalization evoked from forebrain in macaca mulatta. Physiology and Behavior 2: 345–54.

Rolls ET (1992) Neurophysiologic mechanisms underlying face processing within and beyond the temporal cortical visual areas. Bulletin of Biological Science 335: 11–20.

Ross ED (1981) The aprosodias: functional anatomic organization of the affective components of language in the right hemisphere. Archives of Neurology 38: 561–9.

Ross ED (1996) Hemispheric specialization for emotions, affective aspects of language and communication and the cognitive control of display behaviors in humans. In G Holstege, R Bandler, CB Saper (eds) Progress in Brain Research. Oxford: Elsevier Science BV, pp. 583–94.

Ross ED, Mesulam MM (1979) Dominant language functions of the right hemisphere? Archives of Neurology 36: 144–8.

Ross ED, Harney JH, DeLacoste Utamsing, Purdy PD (1981) How the brain integrates affective and propositional language into a unified behavioral function. Archives of Neurology 38: 745–8.

Scott CH (1998) Visualizing fluency. In Scott A. Advance Magazine 8(5): 10.

Shames GH, Florence CL (1980) Stutter-Free Speech: A Goal for Therapy. Columbus OH: Charles Merrill.

Shin LM, Kosslyn SM, McNally RJ, Alpert NM, Thompson WL, Rauch SL, Macklin ML, Pitman RK (1997) Visual Imagery and Perception in Posttraumatic Stress Disorder. A Positron Emission Tomographic Investigation. Arch General Psychiatry 54: 233–41.

Showers MJC, Crosby EC (1958) Somatic and visceral responses from the cingulate gyrus. Neurology 8: 561–5.

Smythies JR (1966) The Neurological Foundations of Psychiatry. New York: Academic Press.

Smythies JR (1968) Biological Psychiatry, a Review of Recent Advances. London: Heinemann Medical Books Limited.

Smythies JR (1970) Brain Mechanisms and Behavior. New York: Academic Press.

Starkweather CW (1991) The language-motor interference in stuttering children. In HFM Peters, W Hulstijn, CW Starkweather (eds) Speech motor and Stuttering. Amsterdam: Elsevier Science Publishers BV, pp. 385–91.

Strauss E, Risser A, Jones MW (1982) Fear responses in patients with epilepsy. Archives of Neurology 39: 626–30.

Szelag E, Garwarska-Kolek D, Herman A, Stasiek J (1993) Brain lateralization and severity of stuttering in children. Acta Neurobiologiae Experimentalis 53: 263–7.

Van Hoesen GW (1995) Anatomy of the medial temporal lobe. Magnetic Resonance Imaging 13: 1047–55.

Walker W (1966) Thalamo-cortical projections. In D Purpura, M Yahr (eds) The Thalamus. New York: Columbia University Press, pp. 18–31.

Warburton E, Wise RJ, Price CJ, Weiller C, Hadar U, Ramsey S, Frackowiak RS (1996) Noun and verb retrieval by normal subjects: studies with PET. Brain 119: 159–79.

Watson M, McElligot JG (1984) Cerebellar norepinepherine depletion and impaired acquisition of specific locomotor tasks in rats. Brain Research 296: 129–36.

Wheatley MD (1944) The hypothalamus and affective behavior in cats: a study of the effects of experimental lesions with anatomic correlations. Archives of Neurological Psychology 52: 296.

Wiesendanger M (1981) Organization of secondary motor areas of the cerebral cortex. In M Wiesendanger (ed.) Handbook of Physiology. Bethesda MD: Williams & Wilkins, pp. 805–51.

Wood F, Stump D, McKeehan A, Sheldon S, Proctor J (1980) Patterns of regional blood flow during attempted reading aloud by stutterers both on and off haloperidol medication: Evidence for inadequate left frontal activation during stuttering. Brain and Language 9: 141–4.

Wu JC, Maguire G, Riley G, Fallon J, LaCasse L, Chin S, Klein E, Tang C, Cadwell S, Lottenberg S (1995) A positron emission tomography [18F] deoxyglucose study of developmental stuttering. Neuroreport 6: 501–5.

Wu JC, Maguire G, Riley G, Lee A, Keator D, Tang C, Fallon J, Najafi A (1997) Increased dopamine activity associated with stuttering. Neuroreport 8: 767–70.

Zimmerman G (1980a) Articulatory dynamics of fluent utterances of stutterers and non-stutterers. Journal of Speech and Hearing Research, 23(1): 95–107.

Zimmerman GN (1980b) Articulatory behaviors associated with stuttering: a cineradiographic analysis. Journal of Speech and Hearing Research 23(1): 108–21.

Zimmerman GN (1980c) Stuttering: a disorder of movement. Journal of Speech and Hearing Research 23(1): 122–36.

Index

Page numbers printed in **bold** type refer to figures

A-B-C paradigm 90
'action circuit' 25
adrenaline 72
adrenocorticotrophic hormone (ACTH) 52
amnesia, anterograde 25, 53
amygdala 12–20, 45
    ablation 13, 15, 18, 52
    cognitive contributions 53
    and conditioned fear 14, 50–4, 97
    connections, *see* amygdala connections
    and emotion 18
    and facial recognition 17–18
    fear and stress 13–14
    location 12
    olfaction 12, 53
    and social behaviour 15–16
    and speech 16
    stimulation 12, 13–14, 45
    synopsis 45
amygdala connections 12–20, 45, 52, 99–105
    anterior cingulate gyrus 18
    auditory 18, 102–3
    basal forebrain 99
    basal ganglia 13, **15**, 17
    brainstem **15**, 16–17, 101
    cingulate gyrus 18, 104
    cortical 102–5
    diencephalon 100–2
    frontal 18, 104
    hippocampus 17, 101–2
    hypothalamus 14, **16**, 20, 100
    hypothalamus-amygdala-hippocampus interface 23

insular 18, 104
larynx 17
midbrain 16
occipital lobes 102–3
periaqueductal grey (PAG) connections **15**, **16**, 17, 18–19
polysensory 103–4
projections to the amygdala 104–5
spinal cord 16
striatum 13, 99
subcortical 99–102
temporal lobes 102–3
thalamus **15**, 100
visual 17, 102
anger 22
anomia 32
anterior area of Ross 11, 40, 45, 63–4, 66
anterior cingulate gyrus (ACG) 27–30, 46
    connections 46
    limbic input 30
    periaqueductal grey (PAG) connections **16**, 18, 30
    and speech 29, 30, 33, 34, 64
    stimulation 27, 28
    synopsis 46
    vocalization 27, 29
anterograde amnesia 25, 53
anticipatory struggle hypothesis 53–4
anxiety
    hypothalamus and 22
    trait *v.* state 67
aphasias 31–2, 33, 35
aprosodia 36–7
archipallium, *see* hippocampus
auditory connections, amygdala 18, 102–3

autism 44
autonomic nervous system, limbic input
    78
avoidance behaviours 49

Bard, P 9
basal forebrain, amygdala connections 99
basal ganglia
    amygdala connections 13, **15**, 17
    conditioning 55–9
    connections 56
    as interface 71
behaviour
    amygdala influence 15–16
    animals *v.* humans 51–2
    and anterior cingulate gyrus 28
    secondary behaviours 50, 82–3, 84
    septal influence 26
    struggle behaviour 82–3, 84
    treatment target 86
behavioural contracts 93–4
belief systems 53–4, 79–80, 84–5, 90, 94
    treatment target 86
blocks, clonic/tonic 49
blood flow
    Broca's area 62
    regional cerebral blood flow (rCBF)
        64, 65, 66, 88–9
    right cerebral hemisphere 47
brain, development 10
brainstem, amygdala connections **15**,
    16–17, 101
Broca's area
    blood flow 62
    cerebellum connections 42
    differences in rCBF in post traumatic
        stress disorder 88–9
    hypoactivation of 64, 66
    limbic inputs 11, 76–8
    major cortical and speech area 39
    and neocerebellum 43, 44, 45, 72
    reversible hypoactivity 67
    and speech 35, 39
    supplementary motor area connec-
        tions 39, 40, 66
    and thalamus 31, 33, 35
Brodman's areas 44

Cannon, WB 9
caudate nucleus
    hypoactivity 68, 70–1

tonically activated neurones (TANs),
    and dopamine 59
cerebellum 42–5, 48, 71
    cerebellar motor system over-
        activation 69, 72
    conditioned responses 42
    connections 48
    development 43
    emotional expression 42, 71
    fear responses 42
    learning 42
    movement 42
    speech and language 33, 34, 43, 71
    stimulation 42
    synopsis 48
    see also neocerebellum
cerebrum
    cerebral dominance, lack of 62
    cerebral motor system over-activation
        69
    regional cerebral blood flow (rCBF)
        64, 65, 66, 88–9
    see also left cerebral hemisphere; right
        cerebral hemisphere
cingulate gyrus 27
    connections to amygdala 104
    mutism 28–9
    stimulation 27
    see also anterior cingulate gyrus
classical conditioning paradigms 49–50
cognitive contributions, amygdala 53
computed tomography 28
conditioning 49–60
    basal ganglia 55–9
    classical conditioning paradigms
        49–50
    conditioned fear 14, 50–4, 96, 97
    conditioned responses, cerebellum 42
    contextual 55
    emotional 55
    hippocampus 24, 54–5
    see also learning
contextual conditioning 55
contracts, behavioural 93–4
control, and the limbic system 10
cortical connections, to amygdala 102–5
cortico-limbic-reticular system 66
counselling 6, 82
courage, client's 86, 90–1

delayed auditory feedback 38

diagnosis 81–5, 95
   implications for 4–5
   information from stutterer 83–4
   severity 81–2, 84–5
   stuttering or normal dysfluency? 81,
      82–4
   traditional 81
diencephalon, amygdala connections
   100–2
diffuse thalamocortical system 30–1
dopamine 53, 57–60, 63, 68, 72, 96–7
Down syndrome 43

electrical stimulation, *see* stimulation
emotion 8
   and the amygdala 18
   'anatomical seat of' 9
   anterior cingulate area 29–30
   cerebellum 42
   'circuit of emotion' 9
   hypothalamus 22
   James–Lange theory 9
   septal influence 26
emotional conditioning 55
emotional expression
   cerebellum 42, 71
   hypothalamus 22
   supplementary motor area (SMA) 39,
      41
emotional facial paralysis 39
emotional imagery 91
emotional memory 55
emotional motor system (EMS) 38–9
emotional reaction 82–3, 84, 95
   treatment target 86
emotional system 4
'empty chair' technique 93
environment, as trigger 1, 2
etiology 1
   historical review of research 8–9
   search for cause of 1–2
extrapyramidal system 56

facial expression 38
facial paralysis, emotional 39
facial recognition, and the amygdala
   17–18
fear
   conditioned 14, 50–4, 96, 97
   reactions to 88
   of stuttering 67–8

fear responses, cerebellum 42
flight-or-fight response 7–8
fluency
   and emotion 8
   induced 56–7, 69
   maintenance of 94
   see also speech and language
Freedom of Fluency 86
frequency counts 5, 83, 84
frontal connections, to amygdala 18, 104

generalization 90–1, 93, 94
Gestalt therapy 91–3
gestures 36
guided visualization 88

haloperidol 62, 63, 96
   side effects 63
heredity 68
hippocampus 3–4, 23–5, 46
   amygdala connections 17, 101–2
   conditioned reflex 24
   conditioning 54–5
   connections 23–5, 46
   hypothalamus-amygdala-hippocam-
      pus interface 23
   learning 25, 54
   limbic involvement 25, 26
   memory 25, 53
   and olfaction 23
   stimulation 24
   synopsis 46
history, etiology research 8–9
hypoactivity
   Broca's area 64, 66, 67
   v. hyperactivity 73
   in left caudate nucleus 68, 70–1
   reversible, in Broca's and Wernicke's
     areas 67
hypothalamus 20–3, 45–6
   ablation 22
   amygdala connections 14, **16**, 20, 100
   anxiety and anger 22
   connections 14, **16**, 20–3, 100
   emotional arousal/expression 22
   hypothalamus-amygdala-hippocam-
     pus interface 23
   and learning 22
   limbic responses 71
   and motivation 22–3
   pituitary gland connections **16**, 21–2

stimulation 21
synopsis 45–6

imaging studies 2–3, 61–73
    summary of results 70
insular connections, to amygdala 18, 104
involuntariness, of stuttering 83

James, William 8–9
James–Lange theory of emotion 9

kindling 73–5, 96, 97
    see also long-term potentiation; stim-
        ulation

Lange, CG 9
language, see speech and language
laryngeal functioning 18–19
larynx, amygdala input to 17
lateral prefrontal cortex 44
lateralization, right hemisphere 65
learning 3, 6
    and the hippocampus 25, 54
    hypothalamus influence 22
    of secondary behaviours 50
    see also conditioning
left cerebral hemisphere
    integration with right hemisphere
        37–8
    and speech 11, 35–6
limbic model 75–80
limbic system 4, 7–8, 9–12
    and control 10
    development 10
    in mammals 9–10
    memory 10
    olfaction 7, 10
    speech 8, 11
    supplementary motor area (SMA) as
        evolutionary extension of 40, 66, 71
    verbalization 11
    vocalization 11
locus of control 5, 6
Locus of Control of Behaviour (LCB) 85,
    94, 95
Locus of Control Scale 5
long-term potentiation (LTP) 74–5, 97
    see also kindling; stimulation

magnetic resonance imaging (MRI) 64
mammillothalamic tract 21

memory 3–4
    emotional 55
    hippocampus 25, 53
    and kindling 74
    and the limbic system 10
    reinforcement 3
mental imagery 87, 89
mesodopamine 72
monotone 8, 29, 38, 41, 63
motivation, hypothalamus influence
    22–3
motor aprosodia 36–7
motor imagery 86–8, 95, 97
    definition 87
    increase in autonomic responses dur-
        ing 88
    v. progressive relaxation 89
movement, and the cerebellum 42
mutism 28–9

neocerebellum 43, 44, 71–2
    speech and language 43, 44, 72
neocortex 43
neuroimaging studies 2–3, 61–73
    summary of results 70
neurotoxins 42
non-emotional stuttering 73–4, 75, 96, 97
noradrenaline 72
nose-brain 7, 10

olfaction
    amygdala 12, 53
    hippocampus 23
    limbic system 7, 10
oro-facial behaviours 56, 57, 59
Orton, S 62

palilalia 33
pantomime 36
Papez, JW 9
paranoia 54
Parkinson's disease 17, 56, 63, 68, 96–7
periaqueductal grey (PAG)
    amygdala connections 15, 16, 17,
        18–19
    anterior cingulate gyrus connections
        16, 18, 30
    as emotional relay centre 19
    vocalization 19
perspectives, clinician v. client 5
PET, see positron emission tomography

pituitary gland, hypothalamus influence
    16, 21–2
play therapy 93
polysensory connections, to amygdala
    103–4
positron emission tomography (PET) 65,
    66–7, 69, 70, 72, 97
post traumatic stress disorder (PTSD)
    88–9
potentiation, *see* long-term potentiation
predisposition to stuttering 1, 2, 68
premotor area 20–1
progressive relaxation, *v.* motor imagery
    89
prosody 36, 66
psychodramas 94
punishment 75
putamen 56, 57

rational emotive behaviour therapy
    (REBT) 90–4
    emotional imagery 91
    Self-Help Form 91, **92**, 95
rational emotive therapy (RET) 54, 85
regional cerebral blood flow (rCBF) 64,
    65, 66, 88–9
relaxation, progressive, *v.* motor imagery
    89
research, future, questions for 96–8
respiration 18–19, 88
reticular formation 24
rhinencephalon 7, 10
rhizotomies 34
right cerebral hemisphere
    abnormal anterior frontal lobe activa-
        tion 62
    blood flow 47
    influence on speech and language
        35–8
    integration with left hemisphere 37–8
    synopsis 47
right hemisphere lateralization 65

Sansert 34
scenario writing 93
schizophrenia 54
secondary behaviours 82–3, 84
    learning of 50
sensory aprosodia 36
septum/septal area 25–6
    savageness after lesions 26

stimulation 47
synopsis 46–7
severity 81–2, 84–5
    Stuttering Severity Instrument 83
single photon emission computed
    tomography (SPECT) 62–3, 64, 70
SMA syndrome 39
smell, *see* olfaction
social behaviour, amygdala influence
    15–16
sources of stuttering 81, 82
specific thalamocortical system 30
SPECT, *see* single photon emission com-
    puted tomography
speech and language
    anterior cingulate gyrus 29, 30, 33, 34,
        64
    aprosodia 36–7
    cerebellum 33, 34, 71
    fluency and emotion 8
    left-hemisphere damage 11, 35–6
    limbic system 8, 11
    monotone 8, 29, 38, 41, 63
    neocerebellum 43, 44, 72
    right cerebral hemisphere 35–8
    supplementary motor area (SMA)
        33–4
    supplementary motor area (SMA) as
        third speech centre 21, 39, 72
    thalamus 31–2, 33, 34, 35
speech naturalness 38
state 66–7
state anxiety 67
stimulation 45
    amygdala 12, 13–14, 45
    cerebellum 42
    cingulate gyrus 27
    hippocampus 24
    hypothalamus 21
    kindling 73–5
    long-term potentiation (LTP) 74–5, 97
    right cerebral hemisphere 47
    septum and septal area 26, 47
    supplementary motor area (SMA) 21,
        31, 39, 40, 41, 47
    thalamus 31, 47
    ventrolateral nucleus 44
stimulus generalization 55
stress mechanism 13–14
stress response 52
striatum

amygdala connections 99
amygdala projections 13
dopamine system 57–8
tonically active neurones (TANs) 57
struggle behaviour 82–3, 84
stuttering-like repetitions 33–4
Stuttering Severity Instrument 83
subcortical connections, to amygdala
        99–102
subcortical structures 7–8
substantia nigra 58, 68
supplementary motor area (SMA) 39–41,
        47–8
    Broca's area connections 39, 40
    connections 39, 48
    emotional expression and 39, 41
    as evolutionary extension of limbic
        system 40, 66, 71
    left v. right 66, 71
    SMA syndrome 39
    speech 33–4
    stimulation 21, 31, 39, 40, 41, 47
    synopsis 47–8
    as third speech centre 21, 39, 72
    and vocalization 21, 40, 41
suprasegmentals 8, 11
surgery 81

tardive dyskinesia 63
temporal lobes 64
thalamocortical systems 30–1
thalamus 30–5, 47
    amygdala connections/projections 15,
        100
    aphasias 31–2, 33
    connections 15, 31, 100
    haemorrhage 32–3
    integrative function 32, 33
    as sensory input centre 30
    specific nuclei of 30, 31
    and speech and language 31–2, 33, 34,
        35
    stimulation 31, 47
    synopsis 47
therapists, characteristics and role 95
tonically active neurones (TANs) 57, 59

toughening techniques 93
trait 66–7
trait anxiety 66–7
trait markers 66–7, 68
Travis, LE 62
treatment 79–80, 86–95
    behavioural contracts 93–4
    bias 6
    emotional imagery 91
    'empty chair' technique 93
    Freedom of Fluency 86
    generalization 90–1, 93, 94
    guided visualization 88
    implications for 5–6
    motor imagery 86–8, 95, 97
    progressive relaxation techniques 89
    rational emotive behaviour therapy
        (REBT) 90–4, 95
    scenario writing 93
trigger, environment as 1, 2
two-factor theory of stuttering 49–50, 55

vagus nerve 16–17, 27
ventral cortical regions 72
ventrolateral nucleus, stimulation 44
verbalization, and the limbic system 11
viscera, and emotions 8–9, 22
visual connections, amygdala 17–18, 102
visual imagery 88–9
    guided visualization 88
visual perception studies 65, 70
vocalization
    anterior cingulate gyrus and 27, 29
    limbic system and 11
    and periaqueductal grey (PAG) 19
    and supplementary motor area (SMA)
        21, 40, 41

Wernicke's area
    cerebellum connections 42
    major cortical and speech area 39
    and neocerebellum 43, 72
    reversible hypoactivity 67
    and speech 35, 39
    and thalamus 31, 33, 35
Williams syndrome 43